SAVE YOUR LIFE

SAVE YOUR LIFE

a handbook for preventing

heart attacks
cancer
strokes

by Lewis Cope

▼ **Published by the Minneapolis Tribune**
425 Portland Av. / Minneapolis, Minn. / 55488

Most of the material in this book has appeared in the Minneapolis Tribune over the last two years. All of it has been brought up to date to include the latest possible information.

First printing

Library of Congress Cataloging in Publication Data

Cope, Lewis, 1934–
 Save your life.

 Includes index.
 1. Heart—Infarction—Prevention. 2. Cancer—Prevention. 3. Cerebrovascular disease—Prevention.
I. Title. [DNLM: 1. Coronary disease—Prevention and control—Popular works. 2. Neoplasms—Prevention and control—Popular works. 3. Cerebrovascular disorders—Prevention and control—Popular works. WG113 C782s]
RC672.C66   613   79-18287

ISBN 0-932272-02-9

Copyright © 1979/Minneapolis Star and Tribune Company

Design / Michael Carroll
Illustrations / John Miller
Compositor / TriStar Graphics

To my daughters Meg, Beth and Amy and my wife Betty

Contents

Heart attacks/
1/ Saving your heart 5
2/ Cholesterol: Good vs. bad 15
3/ High blood pressure: The silent killer 25
4/ Smoking: More than tar and nicotine 33
5/ Weight: You win when you lose 37
6/ Exercise: Benefits and risks 45
7/ Stress: Should you worry about it? 51
8/ Would you recognize a heart attack? 59
9/ CPR: First-aid for heart attacks 65

Cancer/
10/ Defusing the cancer time bomb 73
11/ Smoking and cancer 79
12/ X-rays, drugs and cancer 93
13/ Chemicals, the sun and cancer 103
14/ Your diet and cancer 115
15/ Catching cancer in time 119

Strokes/
16/ Vision blurry? Arm numb? 131

Appendix/
A/ Canadian lifestyle quiz 137
B/ 12 leading causes for death 141
C/ For more information 142

Here's how this book can help you save your life

This book is about three killers — and you. More than that, it's about three killers and what you can do to prevent them from killing you.

The killers are heart attacks, cancer and strokes — the nation's first, second and third leading causes of death. They take the lives of about 1.2 million Americans each year. They are responsible for almost two-thirds of the nation's total deaths.

Much is known — and more continues to be learned — about these diseases and how to prevent them. That's where you come in. In preventive medicine, you're in the driver's seat.

Medical researchers are making great efforts to increase your chances for a long life. But if you don't know about and follow their advice, their efforts will be in vain.

This book pulls together the latest research findings so you can understand the nature of these diseases and learn how to beat the odds against you. It provides practical advice in the form of tips and checklists to help you.

There's more than one reason to follow much of this advice. The causal factors in these diseases are sometimes interrelated, as you will see. Cigarette smoking can cause heart-attack as well as cancer deaths. The diet recommended to help save your heart may protect you from some types of cancer.

Some of the advice about heart attacks and cancer may help prevent other medical problems, too. If you're overweight, you not only risk a heart attack but increase your chances of having diabetes, the nation's sixth highest cause of death. Smoking can lead to crippling and often deadly emphysema, the 12th highest cause of death.

This book can increase your chances for longer life, and make your life more enjoyable, too. If you tend to add pounds, for instance, the chapter on losing weight will tell you how to change the way you eat so you won't have to spend your life on one diet after another. And taking some of the stress out of your life can make you feel better and more vigorous.

There are plenty of choices. It's up to you. This book is designed to help you do what you are willing to do to save your own life.

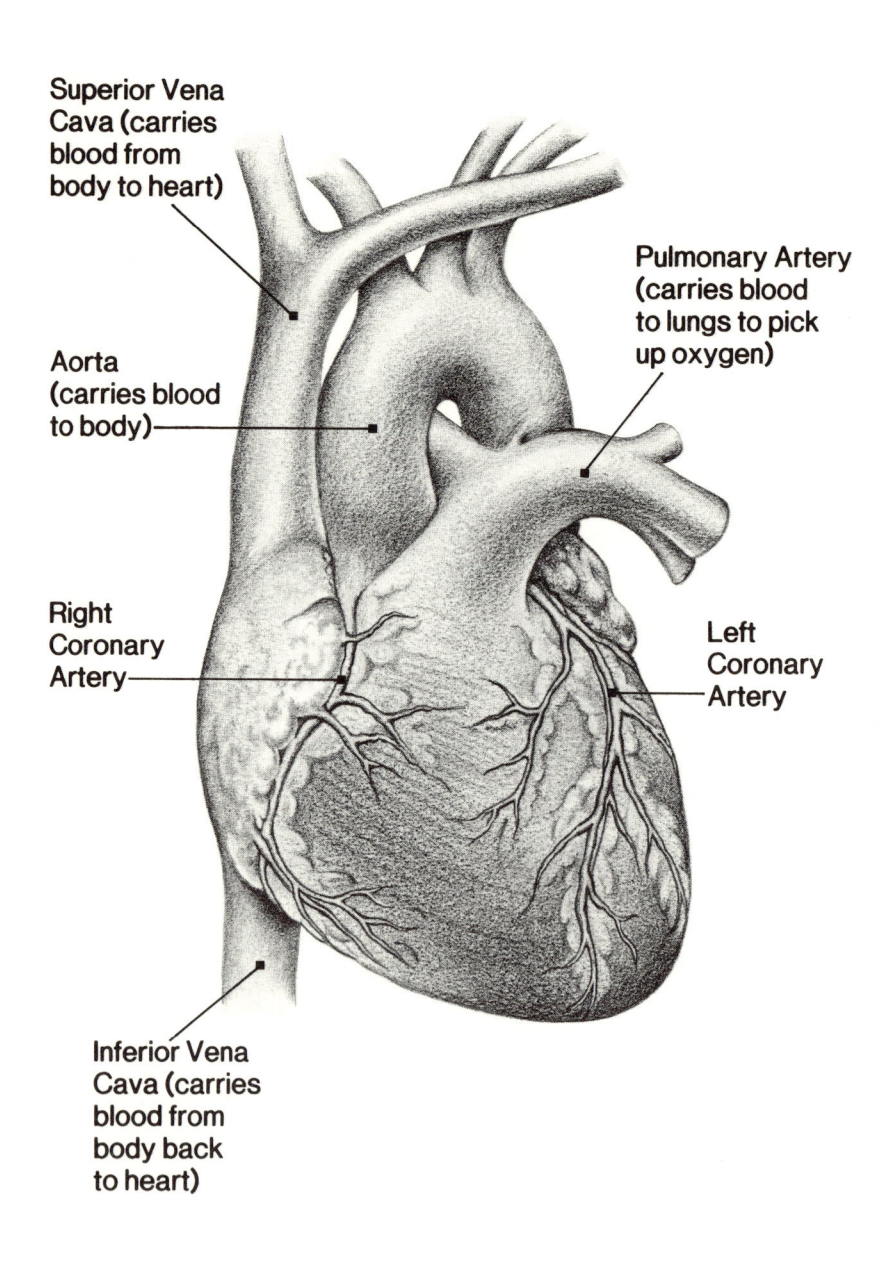

Superior Vena Cava (carries blood from body to heart)

Aorta (carries blood to body)

Right Coronary Artery

Pulmonary Artery (carries blood to lungs to pick up oxygen)

Left Coronary Artery

Inferior Vena Cava (carries blood from body back to heart)

Your heart/
The pump of life

Your heart, which is about the size of your clenched fist, beats 100,000 times each day. By circulating the blood in your body around and around again, it pumps enough to fill a 3,000-gallon tank car every 24 hours.

The right side of the heart sends blood to the lungs to pick up vital, life-giving oxygen that you inhale with each breath of air.

Then the heart's left pumping chamber circulates this blood throughout the tens of thousands of miles of blood vessels in your body. The blood transports not only oxygen to every cell in your body, but other nourishments (such as the building blocks of protein) obtained from the food you eat. And the bloodstream's white blood cells and antibodies stand ready to attack any invading germs or viruses.

The 60,000 miles of blood vessels in a typical-sized adult's body include not only arteries and veins but the smaller arterioles and venules and the cobweb-tiny capillaries.

Your heart muscle, just like the rest of your body, must have life-sustaining blood to survive. That's the job of the two coronary arteries, about the size of soda straws, that branch out through this muscle like spreading trees.

If one of the coronary arteries closes down, blood flow to a section of heart muscle stops. That's a heart attack — the cause of one out of every three deaths in the United States.

1/Saving your heart

Experts in heart-attack prevention are wearing big smiles these days. Here's why:

■ After years of climbing to epidemic proportions, the heart-attack death rate is on a downward path. This comes as Americans are exercising more, smoking less and changing the types of foods they eat.

■ Assuming, as most experts do, that this means prevention efforts are paying off, the welcome surprise is that even moderate changes in lifestyle may pay big dividends against what still is the nation's No. 1 killer.

"The most encouraging thing is how little you apparently have to do to get this much benefit," said Dr. William Kannel of the government's National Heart, Lung and Blood Institute. "Everybody used to say, 'Gee, I'm going to have to give up everything I enjoy.' That's simply not true."

■ Most experts now agree on the "big three" risk factors for heart attacks: diet-related high cholesterol levels, high blood pressure and smoking. Study after study has shown that these are the best indicators of which people are most likely to have heart attacks. But researchers also have gained a much clearer understanding of how three other aspects of lifestyle — exercise, weight and stress — play often indirect but nevertheless important roles.

■ These researchers have developed a picture of how so many factors can be involved in causing heart attacks.

The villains work like this:

Cholesterol — a white, waxy substance — is found in the fatty deposits that can build up, year by year, on the inside walls of the coronary arteries. These fatty deposits can narrow the vessels, much like lime building up in water pipes.

When that happens in a coronary artery, all it takes is a small clot or spasm to close the vessel completely. And this triggers a heart attack by denying nourishing blood to a section of heart muscle.

High blood pressure can pound more cholesterol into these fatty build-ups in the coronary arteries, speeding the narrowing process.

Nicotine in cigarettes makes a smoker's heart work less efficiently so that it needs more oxygen, while carbon monoxide in the inhaled smoke ties up part of the bloodstream's oxygen-transport system.

Weight can affect blood pressure, among other things. Exercise is a big help in keeping weight in line and also may make the heart stronger. Mystery still clouds the role of stress, but it can influence the body's hormonal balance and may trigger a heart attack after other factors have set the stage.

Heart disease: Still a killer

Kannel — a large but trim, soft-spoken man — cautioned against anyone's becoming complacent because of the gains made.

"This is still the leading cause of death," he said. "There's certainly room for a lot of improvement."

Heart attacks took the lives of 637,000 Americans in 1978, with a fourth of the victims under age 65. The toll was down dramatically from 675,000 in 1968.

After allowances are made for the increased population and the growing number of older Americans, the heart-attack death rate has fallen 21 percent since 1968.

"It has occurred in blacks as well as whites, in women as well as men, and in all ages — the elderly as well as the young," Kannel said. "The nation is now experiencing its highest life expectancy."

Kannel said he was very encouraged that the drop in the heart death rate comes as Americans have taken more of the advice of heart experts. Although he said this doesn't prove a cause-and-effect relationship, the drop has occurred as: The consumption of eggs has dropped sharply; margarine has replaced butter on many tables; low-

Risk factors in heart attack

Blood pressure
A man whose blood pressure at systole (the moment the heart contracts) is over 150 has more than two times the risk of heart attack of a man with systolic blood pressure under 120.

Cholesterol
A man with a blood cholesterol measurement of 250 or above has more than twice the risk of heart attack of a man with cholesterol below 194.

Smoking
A man who smokes more than a pack of cigarettes a day has nearly twice the risk of heart attack of a non-smoker.

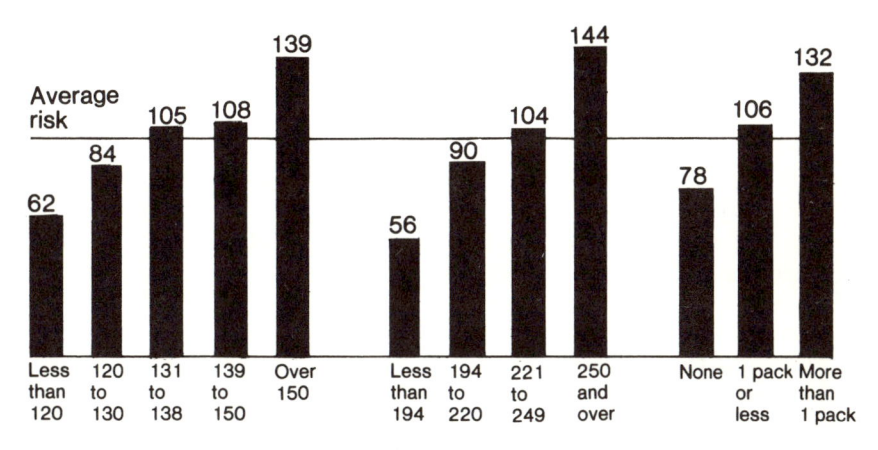

	Average risk									
62	84	105	108	139	56	90	104	144	78	106	132

Blood pressure: Less than 120 | 120 to 130 | 131 to 138 | 139 to 150 | Over 150

Cholesterol: Less than 194 | 194 to 220 | 221 to 249 | 250 and over

Smoking: None | 1 pack or less | More than 1 pack

Source / The Framingham, Mass., Heart Study

fat milk is now commonly used; lean cuts of beef have been found to be plenty juicy.

The experts had predicted that such changes would lower the levels of cholesterol in the bloodstream — and they were right. Surveys show that the average American's cholesterol level has started falling.

Thirty million Americans have quit smoking. Several million have brought their blood pressure down to safe levels with drugs or other treatments since doctors intensified detection efforts about 10 years ago. Joggers have become commonplace, passing other Americans rushing to the tennis courts.

But could the declining death toll be more a reflection of improved care in hospital coronary care units than these changes in lifestyle?

Half of the heart-attack deaths occur before the patient even reaches the hospital, said Dr. Henry Blackburn, the red-bearded director of the Laboratory of Physiological Hygiene at the University of Minnesota, where many pioneering studies in heart-attack prevention have been made.

While improvement in medical care is probably responsible for part of the decrease in the heart-attack death rate, Blackburn said, "my own view is that it could not account for the large change and could not account for the long-term change."

The decrease in the heart death rate began in 1968, but it wasn't until about 1975 that experts decided it was more than a temporary decline. At the American Heart Association's 1978 scientific meeting, not a single expert on a panel discussing the death-rate drop claimed that better medical care was the major factor.

Said Blackburn, pointing to the cholesterol, blood-pressure, treatment and smoking statistics: "When you plug those into the prediction equation, it comes out about what we've observed — about 2 percent a year decrease in (coronary) deaths."

Kannel heads the Framingham Heart Study, in which 5,209 men and women in that Massachusetts city have been followed for 30 years. They have been given complete physical exams and interviews every two years as part of the extensive effort to find out what factors affect their chances of heart attacks.

Kannel's and the Minnesota lab's studies have dramatically shown that the more risk factors a person has, the more likely he or she is to have a heart attack.

"It's a combination of all these influences that results in a joint effect that determines your risk," Kannel explained. "Thus, if you've got everything else going for you, you can get by with smoking to some extent — providing you're willing to put up with emphysema, bronchitis and lung cancer."

Many of us are in trouble

But few Americans have everything going for them.

Blackburn noted that the average level of cholesterol in the United States is still 225 — and it's unusual for anyone in Japan to have a cholesterol level above 180 (milligrams per 100 milliliters of blood).

Japanese traditionally eat little meat, which has kept their blood-cholesterol levels way down. (There are some indications that the Japanese are beginning to eat more meat as they westernize various aspects of their lives, but no detailed data are available.)

In a study completed several years ago, American middle-aged men (age 40 to 59) were found to have a coronary death rate four times that of their Japanese counterparts. The rates for Japanese men and women in other age groups also are very low. Other places with similarly low rates (and low-cholesterol eating patterns) include Yugoslavia, Greece and southern Italy, Blackburn noted.

"That's the potential" for lowering the heart-attack death rate, he said.

Of course, you have to die of something. The Japanese, for example, still die from various causes—but their average longevity is longer because of their relatively low heart death rate.

So some experts speak of preventing "premature" heart attacks.

"But don't ask us to define premature," Blackburn said. "What we really want is for people to die older and healthier. We want their hearts, their legs, their brains to function until it's time to die from whatever."

The Japanese-American differences aren't genetic. When Japanese migrate to the United States, their heart-attack rates increase. Presumably, Blackburn said, this is because they pick up American eating habits.

No one is suggesting that Americans switch their eating style to the traditional Japanese way. In the United States the call is for more limited changes, and that's why Kannel is so pleased with what's happening.

"There have been a lot of people who said, 'Maybe these things work, but the amount of change people would have to make would be unacceptable, too drastic,'" he said. "It's clear that we don't have to subject ourselves to a gastronomic nightmare, or jogging so much that you get bit by a dog. The benefits can be achieved with no threats to the American way of life."

In addition to being one of the top three risk factors for heart attacks, high blood pressure is considered the major cause of strokes. While a heart attack is triggered when blood supply is shut off to a section of heart muscle, a stroke occurs when blood supply is cut off to a section of the brain. The death rate from strokes has been falling in the United States, too.

So your choices of lifestyle can play a big role in when and how you die. As Dr. Robert Hall, medical director of the Texas Heart Institute in Houston, has said: "Ask not what medical science can do to heal your heart, but what you can do to prevent damage to or destruction of your cardiovascular system."

What you can do:

Here, in brief, are nine factors that affect your chances of having a heart attack—*and what you can do to lower your risk:*

The big three...

Cholesterol

Studies have shown that heart attacks are more common among people who have high levels of cholesterol in their blood. The higher the level, the greater the risk.

While this doesn't *prove* that lowering your cholesterol level will decrease the risk of heart attacks, millions of Americans have started modifying their diets as a prudent step.

> *To keep your cholesterol level down, cut back on the amount of saturated fat (the type found in meats and dairy products) and cholesterol (egg yolks are a prime source) in your diet. (See Chapter 2.)*

Blood pressure

Studies show that the higher a person's blood pressure, the greater the risk of a heart attack.

Repeated readings of 140/90 or above indicate high blood pressure. In some cases losing a little weight and cutting back on salt intake may bring the pressure down enough so that treatment with drugs isn't necessary.

In fact, there's a growing theory — not yet proved — that if Americans cut back on salting their food, a lot fewer would have high blood pressure. Federal health officials estimate that 35 million Americans have high blood pressure, including those who take drugs to keep their pressure down to a safe level.

> *Have an annual blood pressure check. Go easy on the salt. (Chapter 3.)*

Smoking

The good news here is that when a cigarette smoker quits, the body quickly clears itself of the nicotine and carbon monoxide that play key roles in heart-attack risk.

Therefore, studies show, the risk of dying from coronary heart disease starts falling almost immediately after a smoker quits, although the risk of dying from lung cancer decreases more slowly. Heart attacks take 60 percent more American lives than *all* types of cancer.

> *Don't smoke. (Tips for quitting in Chapters 4 and 11.)*

These are important, too...

Weight

Being very overweight may directly add to the risk of heart attack by putting an added strain on your heart.

But you don't have to be that overweight for your waistline to be important. Studies indicate that losing excess pounds can help a cholesterol-lowering diet work better. Weight loss also can bring blood pressure down. And being overweight increases a person's risk of developing diabetes. All this helps explain statistics showing that being even moderately overweight can cut life expectancy.

> *If you're overweight, trim back. Then change the way you eat so your weight doesn't bob back up like a Yo-Yo. (Chapter 5.)*

Exercise

Regular, strenuous exercise such as jogging can increase the amount of work your heart can do without excessive strain.

There is growing evidence — but not yet proof — that this will help prevent a heart attack. Moderate exercise may help, too, by controlling weight and in other ways.

Before you buy jogging togs, keep in mind that doctors are concerned about middle-aged people who have been leading sedentary lives for years and then rush into strenuous exercise programs. Since there's a risk of triggering a heart attack in vulnerable people, check with your doctor first.

> *Work out a safe, sensible way to get more exercise. Do things you enjoy doing — so that exercise won't be just a passing phase. (Chapter 6.)*

Stress

It would be nice to say don't worry about this risk factor. But while experts still debate how important stress is in triggering heart attacks, one thing is clear:

If you reduce tension, you're more likely to be able to watch your eating patterns to control your weight and cholesterol levels. Controlling stress often helps a smoker to quit, too.

> *If you stop rushing through life, your life is likely to be longer. (For how to cope with stress, see Chapter 7.)*

You can't change these, but...

Age

The older you are, the more likely you are to have a heart attack if all else is equal. But remember, a fourth of all heart-attack deaths occur in people under age 65.

Sex

Heart attacks are five times more common among men than women before menopause, apparently because of hormonal differences. But the advice above is for women as well as men, said Dr. Blackburn of the University of Minnesota's Laboratory of Physiological Hygiene. Many women have heart attacks — it's just that there is a "five- to 10-year lag" in how the risk factors affect them, Blackburn said.

Heredity

Heredity does play a role, although it's often difficult to separate the roles of family habits and family genes in heart-attack-prone families. It's known that heredity can affect cholesterol levels and a person's susceptibility to high blood pressure. But that doesn't mean there's nothing that can be done about it.

If there is a family history of heart attacks or strokes (a similar process in which blood supply is cut off to a section of the brain rather than the heart), that's all the more reason to keep the six factors at the top of this list under control.

2/Cholesterol: Good vs. bad

The cholesterol story has a new twist.

After years of mounting evidence that this waxy substance is a major villain in the process that leads to heart attacks, a special type of cholesterol that apparently *protects* the heart has been discovered.

But don't strike cholesterol off your list of things to be concerned about. First, the large majority of cholesterol is the "bad guy" type. Second, experts say the discovery of this so-called HDL "good guy" cholesterol actually *helps confirm* the theory that a high-fat, high-cholesterol diet is dangerous to your heart.

So there's more and more reason for you to watch what you eat as a way of keeping your over-all cholesterol level low.

All the answers aren't in yet. But experts have enough are for you to make prudent decisions. Here are the answers to 10 questions you're likely to ask:

What's the evidence for the diet-heart link?

It's circumstantial evidence — but there's a lot of it. And it comes from four directions, tightening a web to strongly implicate what you eat as a major factor determining your vulnerability to a heart attack:

■ As noted in the first chapter, a typical heart attack occurs after cholesterol-rich fatty deposits build up on the inside walls of the coronary arteries. These deposits grow over the years, slowly narrowing these arteries that serve the heart muscle. When a coronary artery becomes very narrowed, a small clot or spasm can close it, shutting off blood to a section of heart muscle to cause a heart attack.

■ Studies in a number of cities across the nation have found that the higher a person's cholesterol level, the greater the statistical chance for a heart attack. For example, other things being equal, a man with a blood cholesterol reading of 250 (milligrams of cholesterol per 100 milliliters of blood) has more than twice the risk of suffering a heart attack as a man with a cholesterol reading below 194.

■ Similar studies comparing people in different countries have shown generally that the higher the consumption of cholesterol-raising foods, the higher the average cholesterol levels in the blood — and the higher the coronary death rate.

While the coronary death rate has been rising in most European countries, it has been falling in the United States and Finland. These are the two nations where the most intensive efforts have been made to encourage people to eat with their hearts in mind.

■ Finally, studies have shown that changes in what you eat can lower your cholesterol level. It's not enough to just cut back on cholesterol-rich foods such as egg yolks, since the body also makes its own cholesterol. You also have to cut back on the consumption of saturated fats (typically animal fats), since this type of fat tends to keep the body's over-all cholesterol level up.

(Your body needs some cholesterol — you just don't want to have too much. Cholesterol forms part of the protective cover of nerves, and it's the starting substance from which some vital hormones, including sex hormones, grow.)

What about that type of cholesterol that *protects* the heart?

This "good guy cholesterol," bound to a heavy protein that carries it through the bloodstream, is called high-density lipoprotein (HDL). Some people have more HDL cholesterol than others. The more the better, the new studies indicate.

Researchers believe that HDL serves as a sort of "garbage truck," picking up excess cholesterol off the walls of the coronary and other arteries, then carrying it to the liver, where it's broken down.

On first look, it might appear that this discovery knocks a big hole in the theory that a low-cholesterol, low-fat diet can reduce your chance of having a heart attack.

"Not at all," explained Dr. Henry Blackburn of the University of Minnesota's Laboratory of Physiological Hygiene, where many of the

Setting the stage for a heart attack

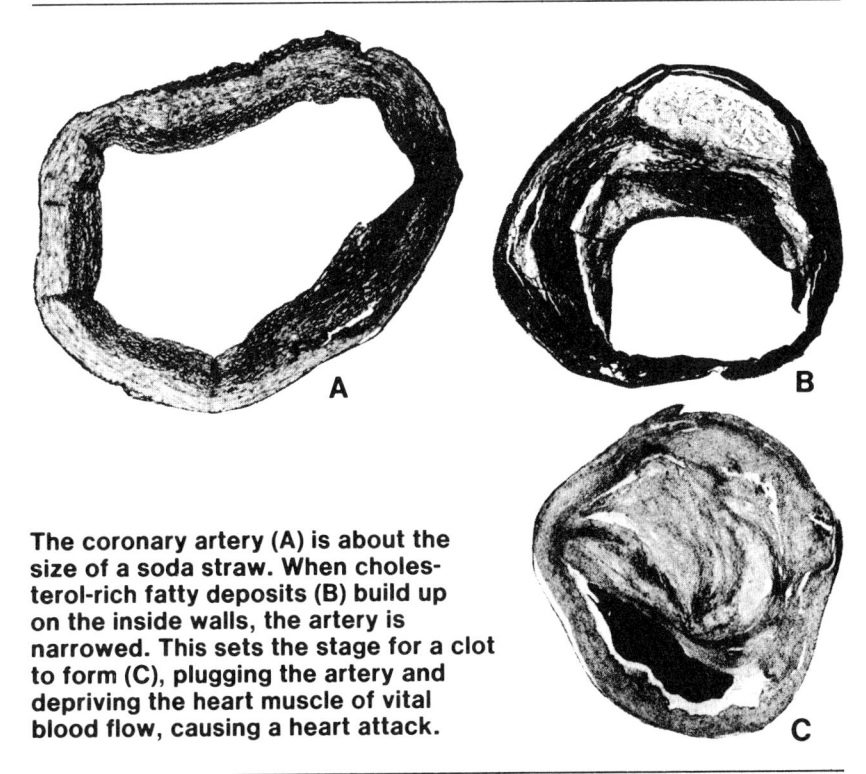

The coronary artery (A) is about the size of a soda straw. When cholesterol-rich fatty deposits (B) build up on the inside walls, the artery is narrowed. This sets the stage for a clot to form (C), plugging the artery and depriving the heart muscle of vital blood flow, causing a heart attack.

Source / American Heart Association

pioneering studies on cholesterol have been done. "It's added knowledge," he said.

For example, doctors have been puzzled because sometimes people with very low levels of cholesterol in their blood had heart attacks. And vice-versa.

"It helps us explain those small departures" from the cholesterol theory, Blackburn said. You shouldn't stop worrying about cholesterol because some of it is good, he emphasized.

His laboratory checked blood samples of several thousand residents in Richfield, Minn. In 80 percent of the cases the HDL levels were average and therefore didn't affect the risk classification of the individual based on total cholesterol.

In 10 percent of the cases the person was better off than otherwise would have been expected, thanks to a high HDL level. Just the opposite was true in another 10 percent of the cases.

HDL cholesterol also may help explain how some other healthy habits affect a person's risk of having a heart attack.

For example, strenuous exercise such as jogging tends to increase the level of HDL in a person's blood. HDL levels also tend to rise when people quit smoking or lose weight. In these cases the level of this "good cholesterol" tends to go up, and the level of the dangerous kind goes down.

But even if the HDL levels are up, it's important to keep the level of the rest of the cholesterol as low as possible, Blackburn said.

Watching what you eat "is just as important as it ever was," he emphasized.

In most people, HDL accounts for only about 20 percent of the total cholesterol in the bloodstream.

Speaking of cholesterol in general, is it necessary to have a person's cholesterol level measured before trying to lower it?

No. The dietary steps at the end of this chapter are recommended for all.

Some doctors do take blood samples from their patients to find out precisely how high their cholesterol levels are. This is done particularly, but not exclusively, if there's a history of heart trouble in the family that may indicate a genetic tendency to elevated blood-cholesterol levels.

Some doctors also test for levels of other fats (such as triglycerides) in the blood, although most studies indicate that cholesterol is the fatty substance that most people should be concerned about. Now some doctors also are starting to check for HDL as well.

So the discovery of HDL's protective role may improve a doctor's ability to assess your individual risk. It also provides one more good reason to quit smoking or shed excess pounds. But, Blackburn said, in no way does HDL make the diet-determined cholesterol less important.

Is there a safe level of cholesterol to have in the blood?

Generally the lower the better, studies indicate, at least down to about 180 (which is very low). The average American adult's cholesterol level is now about 225, although there's variation from person to person depending on genetic factors as well as diet. One of every five American adults has a level of 250 or above.

Even if one member of a family is blessed with a low cholesterol level, the entire family should have a prudent, low-fat eating pattern for the benefit of the other family members, Blackburn said.

How much can a person reduce his or her cholesterol level by following the prudent diet steps listed at the end of this chapter?

By about 10 percent, experts say.

On the average, that would reduce a person's statistical risk of having a heart attack by 24 percent. The precise risk reduction would vary somewhat from case to case, however, depending primarily on what level the person started from. All this assumes the cholesterol-lowering theory is correct; some critics still challenge it.

Why?

The critics question the idea that a *change* in a person's cholesterol level will really help.

One possibility is that once cholesterol deposits have begun to be laid down in the coronary arteries, it might be too late for a change to help.

However, experiments in a number of different types of animals have shown that fatty, cholesterol-rich buildups in the coronary arteries can be reversed with a change in diet. The HDL "good cholesterol," in fact, may be what removes some of the cholesterol from the artery walls.

Then why haven't some experiments with cholesterol-lowering drugs provided clear evidence that the risk of a heart-attack can be lowered?

Experts note that these drugs had been used primarily in middle-aged people with very high cholesterol levels, many of whom also smoked and had other heart "risk factors" working against them.

"It's unrealistic to think that lowering one risk factor alone at such an advanced age would have any dramatic effect," Blackburn said.

Still, he said, the evidence indicates that it helps anyone to lower cholesterol levels, regardless of age — it just helps more if other risk factors also are lowered.

But even if it turns out that it's too late for some to be helped by changes in their diet, he said, parents can be showing by example how their youngsters should eat to protect their hearts.

"I think there's sufficient reason that it's worthwhile to counsel everyone to make changes in their diet," he said.

In some surveys in this country, those who report they eat a lot of meat and other cholesterol-raising foods haven't been found to have higher cholesterol levels than other Americans. Why not?

"Some of us think it's because everybody (in the United States) is eating too much of the wrong thing, so we don't have the contrast we need to see these things," said Dr. William Kannel of the National Heart, Lung and Blood Institute.

Blackburn said that individual heredity variations are enough to confuse such studies. But even if you have a genetic tendency to higher cholesterol levels, he said, you can reduce their level by dietary changes. Such individuals may not get as low as someone else, but they can get lower than they are now.

Is there any risk in changing to the type of eating pattern being recommended as "prudent" by the American Heart Association and other experts?

Blackburn noted that the suggested changes for Americans are along the lines of what's already being practiced in many other countries. The prudent diet still allows a lot of meaty meals, but with an emphasis on smaller portions and leaner cuts.

As experts try to learn more and more about HDL "good cholesterol," at least one study has found that moderate drinking (one or two highballs a day) may raise the level of HDL. Is drinking good for the heart?

Experts are quick to point out that much more has to be learned about HDL — and that there is also evidence that heavy drinking can damage the heart muscle directly.

What you can do:

Here's how various types of fat in the diet affect the cholesterol level in your blood:

■ **Saturated fats** tend to raise the level of cholesterol in the blood, increasing your heart risk. These are fats that usually harden at room temperature. They are found in most animal products, including meats and dairy products. But there also are saturated vegetable fats in many solid and hydrogenated shortenings, and in coconut oil, cocoa butter and palm oil.

■ **Polyunsaturated fats** tend to lower the level of cholesterol in the blood. They are usually liquid oils of vegetable origin. Examples are safflower, soybean and corn oil.

■ **Monosaturated fats** neither raise nor lower cholesterol levels. Examples are peanut oil and olive oil.

■ **Eating cholesterol** itself can raise the level of cholesterol in your blood. Cholesterol-rich foods include egg yolks and organ meats (such as liver), and shellfish. There's also cholesterol in red meat.

The prudent way to eat

The basic approach of the prudent diet is to cut back in total fat consumption (as a good way of controlling weight) as well as to watch the kinds of fats consumed with your cholesterol level in mind.

Sources for the suggestions in this "What you can do" section are the American Heart Association and Patricia Ashman of the University of Minnesota School of Public Health.

To control the amount and type of fat you eat:

■ Use fish, chicken, turkey and veal for more of your meat meals. Use beef, lamb, pork and ham less frequently, and keep the portions moderate.

■ Choose lean cuts of meat. Trim visible fat and discard the fat that cooks out of the meat.

■ Limit your use of fatty "luncheon" and "variety" meats such as sausages, salami, frankfurters and liverwurst, all of which have high fat content.

■ Instead of butter and other cooking fats that are solid or completely hydrogenated, use liquid vegetable oils and margarines that are high in polyunsaturated fats. Safflower oil is the most polyunsaturated. Following it in descending order are sunflower, soybean, corn and cottonseed oils.

■ Instead of whole milk and cheeses made from whole milk and cream, use skimmed milk, skimmed-milk cheeses, low-fat cottage cheese and yogurt. Try sherbets instead of ice cream.

■ Eat more vegetables and fruits rather than meat. Make vegetables more tempting by adding herbs and spices.

■ Add variety to your meal planning by having some meatless meals. Some examples are spaghetti with meatless sauce, meatless chili and vegetable soup.

To control your intake of cholesterol-rich foods:

■ Eat no more than three egg yolks a week, including eggs used in cooking, the American Heart Association recommends. Egg whites and the low-cholesterol egg substitutes can be used.

■ Limit your use of shrimp and organ meats.

How to protect your family while cooking

Even lean meat has fat in it. The American Heart Association offers these suggestions for reducing the saturated fat in the meat you do eat:

■ Use a rack to drain off the fat when broiling, roasting or baking. Instead of basting with drippings, keep meat moist by pouring cooking wine over it.

■ Cook a day ahead of time any stews, boiled meat, soup stock or other dishes in which fats cook into the liquid. After the food has been refrigerated, the hardened fat can be removed from the top.

■ Make gravies after the fat has hardened and can be removed from the liquid.

■ Broil, rather than pan-fry, meats such as hamburger, lamb chops, pork chops and steak.

Don't be misled

■ Buttermilk, despite its name, is a good thing to drink. It's normally made with low-fat milk, and its name comes from the process used to make it rather than any indication that it contains butter.

■ Be leery of imitation dairy products. Most contain coconut oil, which is highly saturated.

Eating smart while eating out

Here are suggestions for eating out, from the American Heart Association Cookbook (available in bookstores):

■ Get into the habit of saying no to cream soups, fried foods, casseroles and other mixed dishes, creamed foods, gravies, cheeses, ice creams, puddings, cakes, pies and similar desserts.

■ If you can, choose from:

First course: Clear soup, tomato juice, fruit cup.

Main dish: Fish or chicken (baked or broiled without butter); sliced turkey or veal; London broil (flank steak) without gravy; fruit, gelatin or fish salad (watch amount and type of dressing); vegetable plate (if butter hasn't been added.)

Dessert: Fruit; sherbet; gelatin; unfrosted angel food cake.

Checking your foods for fat content

Ingredients of commercial baked products and other processed foods are listed on food labels, in order of their quantity in the product. So the higher that a fat is on the list, the more of it that's likely to be in the food. Remember, oils high in saturated fats include palm oil, coconut oil and cocoa butter. The next section gives more information on some fats and oils you may see listed on labels.

Fats and oils: How much, in what?

Ounce for ounce (or gram for gram), saturated fats are twice as effective in raising blood cholesterol levels as polyunsaturates are in lowering it.

This table from the American Heart Association Cookbook shows the amount of cholesterol (in milligrams) and fatty acids (in grams) contained in a tablespoon of each item:

	cholesterol	saturated	mono-unsaturated	poly-unsaturated
Butter	35	6.0	4.0	trace
Lard	13	5.0	6.0	1.0
Tub margarine				
liquid safflower	0	1.5	2.5	6.7
liquid corn oil	0	2.0	3.6	5.3
Stick Margarine				
liquid corn oil	0	2.1	4.6	4.1
Stick or tub margarine				
with partially hydrogenated or hardened fat	0	2.4	6.2	2.0
Imitation (diet) margarine	0	1.0	1.8	2.5
Mayonnaise	8	2.0	2.0	6.0
Vegetable shortening				
(hydrogenated)	0	3.0	6.0	3.0
Corn oil	0	2.0	4.0	8.0
Cottonseed oil	0	4.0	3.5	6.5
Safflower oil	0	1.5	2.0	10.5
Sesame oil	0	2.0	6.0	6.0
Soybean oil	0	2.0	3.5	8.5
Soybean oil (lightly hydrogenated)	0	2.0	7.0	4.8
Sunflower oil	0	1.6	3.9	8.5
Olive oil	0	2.8	7.0	3.9
Peanut oil	0	2.0	10.0	2.0
Coconut oil	0	13.0	1.0	trace

3/High blood pressure: The silent killer

When Walter Mondale went in for his annual physical checkup in 1970, Dr. Milton M. Hurwitz of St. Paul routinely wrapped a blood-pressure cuff around Mondale's arm.

The doctor's diagnosis, after confirmation on repeat examinations: Mondale is one of the estimated 35 million Americans who have high blood pressure.

High blood pressure is a silent killer, normally causing no identifiable symptoms. Left untreated, it's a major cause of heart attacks, strokes and kidney failure. Any repeated readings of 140/90 or higher are a concern.

The discovery that Mondale, then a senator, had high blood pressure didn't keep him from becoming vice president of the United States.

And there is no reason it should have, as the comments by many doctors made clear before his nomination.

Mondale takes five pills a day that keep his blood pressure, which had been only moderately high even at his top reading of 150/102, down to normal. People like Mondale are still considered to have high blood pressure, and thus are included in the 35-million estimate, since their pressure would shoot up if they stopped their medication.

But how about the rest of us?

What worries health officials is the millions of other Americans who have high blood pressure and either don't realize it or have stopped taking their drugs for one reason or another.

"With proper treatment, a person can bring his or her blood pressure down and can look forward to living a full, normal life," says the National Heart, Lung and Blood Institute, which is leading a national effort to detect and treat high blood pressure.

But Graham Ward, coordinator of the institute's high blood pressure control program, said surveys indicate that fewer than half of the 35 million Americans with high blood pressure have it under control.

Sometimes a person actually feels better not taking a prescribed medication, because of side effects such as occasional headaches and diarrhea. While doctors say these side effects usually can be limited or prevented by finding the right amount of the right drug, it's still difficult for some people to shell out money for a drug to treat a symptomless ailment. (Mondale's doctor said the vice president has no side effects from his medication.)

The medical term for high blood pressure, hypertension, adds to the problem.

"People confuse hypertension with nervous tension," Ward said. Hypertension simply means that the pressure of the blood against the walls of the arteries is too high, but he said some people mistakenly take their medication only when they feel tense. Or only when they "feel bad," which is no criterion to use for a symptomless ailment.

But doesn't stress have *something* to do with high blood pressure?

"Any kind of emotions, positive or negative, or physical activity can bring blood pressure up temporarily, but then it falls down," Ward noted.

The concern is about blood pressure that stays high. Asked if stress can cause this, Ward said:

"We don't know. If you look at occupations that appear to be particularly stressful, such as firemen and policemen, you don't find it. There is only one occupational group that has been found to have an increased level — air traffic controllers."

So a very calm person can have high blood presssure. Again, the only way to be sure is to have your blood pressure checked periodically.

The role of salt

Drugs aren't always necessary to bring blood pressure down to a safe level. Often if a person is overweight, taking off the excess pounds will bring the blood pressure under control. Cutting back on salt in the diet helps others.

Blood pressure

	Systolic/Diastolic	Added life expectancy Men	Women
Age 35	120/80	41½ yrs.	No data compiled
	130/90	37½	
	140/95	32½	
	150/100	25	
Age 45	120/80	32 yrs.	37 yrs.
	130/90	29	35½
	140/95	26	32
	150/100	20½	28½
Age 55	120/80	23½ yrs.	27½ yrs.
	130/90	22½	27
	140/95	19½	24½
	150/100	17½	23½

Source/Metropolitan Life Insurance Co.

In some parts of the world where the people eat meager amounts of salt, high blood pressure is relatively rare. Among Americans, who eat a lot of salt, high blood pressure is common. Of course, other factors differ from country to country, too. But the discovery of these differences, along with some animal experiments, have led to this theory:

Some people may be genetically susceptible to high blood pressure. For them, eating a lot of salt may trigger the problem. But the only way to find out who is vulnerable would be to have each person eat a lot of salt to see if it triggers high blood pressure.

"The salt question is probably the least well understood of things that have to do with hypertension," said Dr. Mary Jane Jesse, director of the heart disease division of the National Heart, Lung and Blood Institute.

"People will run around and say that high consumption of salt will cause hypertension. That is not known. What we know is that with populations where very little salt is eaten, the incidence of hypertension is low."

But she said prudence dictates that you don't have to wait for the results from research now under way to start playing it safe.

"When I talk to a family or to patients, I ask them how much salt they eat," she said. "I try to get an idea whether they cook with salt, and do they use extra salt at the table. I tell them to begin to cut back, preferably by taking the salt shaker off the table."

Is salt that's added at the table more important than salt used in cooking?

"No, salt is salt is salt," she said, but many people do find it easier to cut back on the table salt.

Pressure in your plumbing

Why is high blood pressure so dangerous?

"If you put a high head of pressure in any plumbing, sooner or later you're going to have trouble with it," said Jesse.

Blood pressure can contribute to the narrowing of the heart's coronary arteries in two ways.

First, the high pressure may slightly damage the arteries, much as a garden hose wears out more quickly if you're constantly using it at high pressure. This damage makes the soda-straw-size arteries more vulnerable to the build-up of fatty deposits.

Second, the high pressure tends to push more of the blood's cholesterol into these fatty buildups. When a coronary artery becomes narrowed by these deposits, this increases the danger that a small clot or spasm will completely close the artery. If that happens the flow of nourishing blood to a section of heart muscle is cut off — and that's a heart attack.

High blood pressure, depending on how high it is, may double a typical person's chance of having a heart attack. But if that person has both high blood pressure and a high level of cholesterol in the blood because of the type of foods he or she eats, the risk can be several times normal.

What you should know:

How often should blood pressure be checked?

Once a year for adults.

Does this mean I have to see my doctor to have my blood pressure checked?

No.

■ Many city and county health departments offer blood pressure tests, usually without charge.

■ In some communities, firemen who serve as paramedics will do free testing at fire stations when they aren't out on emergency runs.

■ Another good place to try is the company medical office or nurse where you work.

■ Booths sometimes are set up in shopping centers for free blood-pressure testing.

■ While physicians usually charge when they see a patient, some doctors have their nurses take blood-pressure readings without charge. You can phone to find out what your doctor's policy is.

What are the symptoms of high blood pressure?

Don't count on symptoms to warn you.

Many people don't have any. If there are symptoms, they're things like occasional headaches, nosebleeds and dizziness — things that have many different causes. The only way to know is to have your blood pressure checked.

How high does blood pressure have to be to be considered high blood pressure?

Anything consistently at or above 140/90 is considered at least marginally high, and 160/95 is definitely high, said Ward of the National Heart, Lung and Blood Institute. (The estimate of 35 million Americans with high blood pressure is based on a person's receiving treatment or having a pressure above 160/95.)

If your blood pressure is only marginally high, your doctor may monitor it closely for a while to see if it creeps up. Your doctor also may suggest that you lose weight, if you're overweight, or cut back on salt intake since both of these approaches often can lower blood pressure.

Doesn't blood pressure increase with age?

It tends to do so among Americans, but not in many other countries. Diet and other factors may be responsible for this American experience. In any case, most experts say, age is no excuse for not treating high blood pressure, although it may be taken into consideration in marginal cases.

Can blood pressure be too low?

Not as long as you don't feel faint or ill, most experts say. "It just means you're going to live a long time unless you get hit by a truck," Ward said.

How long does it take to have blood pressure checked?

One to two minutes.

How is blood pressure measured?

An inflatable rubber cuff, connected to a pressure gauge, is wrapped around the upper arm. Enough air is pumped into the cuff to cut off circulation.

As the air is gradually released, the person taking the reading listens with a stethoscope for the first sound of blood rushing through the artery. The reading on the gauge at that moment is the systolic pressure — the pressure as the heart pumps.

More air is released from the arm cuff. When the sound disappears, the cuff is no longer having an effect. The pressure reading at that moment is the diastolic pressure — the pressure of blood in the artery when the heart is at rest.

What do the numbers of a blood-pressure reading mean?

The top, or largest number, is the systolic pressure, with the heart contracting to pump blood out. The bottom number is the diastolic measure.

The numbers themselves mean how high, in millimeters, the pressure will force up a column of mercury. For example, 120/80 means that when the heart is pumping, the pressure will push up a column of mercury 120 mm; when the heart is at rest the pressure through the artery will still push the column of mercury up 80 mm.

Which number is most important — the top one or bottom one?

Both are important.

What if blood pressure is high one day but normal another?

"Blood pressure is not like the pressure in a tire, which is the same all the time," Ward said. It goes up and down during the day, influenced by physical activity and other things.

Unless it's very high, there's not much concern about a single-day above-average reading. There are fluctuations of blood pressure for various reasons, and the main worry is for sustained high readings. But you may be asked to come back for periodic rechecks.

Should children have their blood pressure checked?

More and more doctors are doing it, and public health officials are encouraging it. Only a few children have blood pressures high enough to require treatment with drugs, but this allows borderline cases to be identified early so that they can be closely monitored into adulthood.

Family record of blood pressure readings

Name	Date	Reading	Approx. weight	Any comments
		/		
		/		
		/		
		/		
		/		
		/		
		/		
		/		
		/		
		/		
		/		
		/		
		/		
		/		
		/		
		/		
		/		
		/		
		/		
		/		

4/Smoking: More than tar and nicotine

When Nick Clark blew up a plastic balloon, it was the beginning of the end for his 2½-pack-a-day smoking habit.

The balloon was hooked up to a small machine that measures concentrations of carbon monoxide, an odorless and colorless gas.

The dial shot up to 28, showing that the concentration of carbon monoxide in his exhaled breath was 28 parts per million. This, in turn, meant that 5 percent of the red blood cells in Clark's body were tied up carrying carbon monoxide rather than oxygen.

"I knew that carbon monoxide is a poisonous gas," Clark said, "but I don't think smokers normally think about it."

But two weeks later — still thinking about it — he quit smoking. While the balloon test was just one of the reasons he quit, it provides dramatic evidence of how smoking affects the heart.

Tar and nicotine content of cigarettes has received the greatest public attention. But carbon monoxide is one of the major reasons that cigarette smokers have an increased risk of suffering heart attacks, typically twice the risk of a nonsmoker.

The inhaled nicotine tends to make the heart beat harder and somewhat faster (but less efficiently), which increases the demand of the heart for oxygen.

At the same time, the carbon monoxide in inhaled smoke gets into the bloodstream and binds extremely tightly with red blood cells that should be carrying oxygen. This reduces the amount of oxygen the blood can carry.

"The smoker's heart needs more but gets less oxygen than usual, so a large strain is put on the heart," explained Eileen Rotman, an expert on helping smokers quit.

A heart put under this stress apparently is more susceptible to the other processes that lead to heart attacks. And smoking may contribute to them, too.

Some researchers believe that carbon monoxide can damage the coronary arteries, making them more vulnerable to cholesterol deposits. Researchers also have found that smoking affects the body's blood-clotting system. The typical heart attack occurs when a coronary artery, already narrowed by cholesterol and other fatty deposits, is completely closed by a clot or spasm.

Clark, who was 38 when he gave up cigarettes in 1977, had been smoking for 23 years.

He took the balloon test again — just for fun — to mark the first anniversary of his quitting cigarettes. The machine's needle barely budged. (Everyone inhales a little carbon monoxide from car exhausts and other combustion processes.)

"You're a confirmed nonsmoker now," said Rotman, who had given Clark the original balloon test as part of her Unsmoke program. She holds Unsmoke sessions at several hospitals and clinics to help smokers quit, and also is a member of the faculty at the University of Minnesota's School of Public Health.

When you think of the health effects of smoking, lung cancer (caused by the tar in smoke) is likely to lead your list.

But cigarette smoking, as one of the major risk factors for heart attack, is responsible for 20 to 25 percent of all heart-attack deaths, a number of researchers have concluded. Twenty percent of the 637,000 Americans who died of heart attacks in 1978 figures out to more than 125,000 lives. By comparison, 92,000 Americans died of lung cancer that year.

But the rewards from stopping smoking are great.

Within 24 hours after you stop smoking, the levels of nicotine and carbon monoxide in the body are down to near-normal levels.

"The risk of dying from (coronary) heart disease is reduced almost immediately after cessation of smoking, while the risk of dying from lung cancer decreases more slowly," notes a report by Department of Health, Education and Welfare smoking experts.

Studies indicate that it takes a few years after quitting for the full benefit to the heart to be achieved. And while the benefit to the lung is slower, quitting is still important. Other studies show that 10 years after giving up cigarettes, over-all mortality rates reach near-normal levels.

The balloon test is no magic solution, Rotman emphasized. It's just one of many possible ways of helping smokers reach a decision to stop.

"The most important is for smokers to realize that they have choices," she said.

Thirty million Americans have quit smoking since the U.S. surgeon general's first report on smoking and health was issued in 1964. But in considering whether to smoke or not, Rotman said, factors other than health should be considered, too. For example, think of the money saved: She calculated that Clark had "unsmoked 18,000 cigarettes" over the past year by quitting, saving $600.

Studies indicate that cigarettes low in tar and nicotine content are *less* of a health risk, but giving up cigarettes entirely is by far the safest thing to do. However, for people who have tried to quit abruptly without success, low-tar-and-nicotine cigarettes may provide a stepping stone to cessation.

"To leave a smoker with the feeling that all you can do is quit overnight is unrealistic," Rotman said.

She suggests a five-week plan for these smokers: Never smoke the same brand twice. Continually move down to cigarettes lower in tar and nicotine, trying to cut down on the number of cigarettes smoked daily, too. By the end of the five weeks, the smoker should be puffing on cigarettes with 2 mg or less tar. This will make it much easier to quit.

(Cigarette brands low in tar and nicotine tend be lower in carbon monoxide output, too, but not in every case. And since the cigarette packs don't list carbon monoxide content, a smoker has no way of knowing how much of a risk his or her particular brand poses.)

A caution: While pipe and cigar smoking is sometimes considered relatively "safe" (there are still some health risks), be careful if you're switching from cigarettes to these other forms of tobacco. Pipes and cigars aren't safe if you inhale the smoke.

In addition to the heart risk, some studies have found an increased risk of strokes (in which blood supply is cut off to a section of the brain) among smokers. Emphysema, a disabling and potentially deadly lung disease, is clearly linked to smoking. And several types of cancer in addition to lung malignancies are caused by smoking.

Studies have linked smoking to heart attacks in women as well as men, and there are three special health risks that women smokers should consider:

■ **The birth control pill** and smoking don't mix. "Pill users who also smoke are three times more likely to die of a heart attack or other circulatory disease than women who do not use the pill and do not smoke," says a report by the Food and Drug Administration.

■ **Smoking during pregnancy** increases the risk of miscarriages and death in early infancy.

■ **Babies born to mothers who smoke** tend to be smaller; since the smoking doesn't affect the duration of pregnancy, it apparently interferes directly with growth. "Studies of long-term growth and development give evidence that smoking during pregnancy may affect physical growth, mental development and behavioral characteristics of children at least up to the age of 11," notes the U.S. surgeon general's 1979 Smoking and Health report. British and Israeli studies found that smoking mothers' babies are more likely to be hospitalized for bronchitis or pneumonia during their first year of life.

5/Weight: You win when you lose

"About 20 percent of the adults in the United States are overweight to a degree that may interfere with optimal health and longevity. After age 40, this figure jumps to a startling 35 percent." — National Institutes of Health

The most perplexing thing about trying to lose weight is the Yo-Yo effect.

The typical overweight American has lost plenty of pounds — plenty of times — only to watch the weight come back up each time.

The idea of behavior-modification weight reduction is to prevent this by changing the *way* a person eats, not just *what* he or she eats, so that the change will be permanent after the dieting period is over. And keeping the weight off is what's important to good health.

"Eat to live, rather than live to eat," suggests Vikki Mullenbach, director of the Changing Weighs program at Metropolitan Medical Center in Minneapolis. The idea, she said, is to eat amply to satisfy hunger, but to find other ways of relieving tension or whatever is triggering overeating.

It's Changing *Weighs*, not *weights*, because it emphasizes the way a person eats. If you're interested in losing weight, here's a four-step do-it-yourself plan based on this approach:

Step 1: Your "Eating Diary"

Find out *how* and *why* you're consuming more calories than you need. Keep an "eating diary" for a week before you start trying to reduce.

Jot down in a notebook everything you eat or drink — with the time, place, how long you take to eat either the meal or snack, what else you may be doing at the time, your mood (happy, depressed, angry, etc.) and how hungry you are.

(For hunger, use a scale or 0 to 5, with 3 ideal. You don't want to get too hungry before you eat; that may cause you to overeat or sneak a snack.)

You may be surprised how much you've been eating without thinking about it. Or without really being hungry. But the main idea is to find your "trouble spots" for overeating. For example, you may automatically snack while watching TV, or overeat when you're tired.

Step 2: Fit your actions to your needs

After you identify why and how you eat — from both the diary and anything else you know about your eating patterns — use the list of suggestions at the end of the chapter. Check the appropriate boxes for the tips *you* think will help *you*.

Continue keeping the food diary for a few weeks, but in abbreviated form, as you cut back on your eating to shed excess pounds. Concentrate on the "trouble spots" you have found. For example, if you find you snack when tired or angry, just keep track of what you eat and your mood at the time.

Step 3: Your point system

Set up a system of points based *not* on how many pounds you take off, but how well you follow the changes in eating behavior that you've selected. Each day award yourself five points for each checked suggestion that you have followed, plus 25 bonus points if you've followed every checked suggestion on your list.

When you accumulate a self-selected number of points, treat yourself to a reward. Maybe new clothes (with a smaller waistline). Or a trip. Or something else you want.

Step 4: Steady as you go

After you're down to your desired weight, the hope is that you will have changed the way you eat. But don't leave it to hope. Keep this list and go back over it once a month so you will continue eating in a sensible pattern.

How important is weight to health?

For a person who's very overweight — 30 percent over normal — the extra pounds can put a strain on the heart that may increase the risk of a heart attack.

For a person only moderately overweight, most experts now agree that if such a direct risk exists it's small. But excess weight works in so many indirect ways, by affecting other heart risk factors, that weight is still very important:

■ An overweight person is more likely to have high blood pressure, a major cause of heart attacks, strokes and kidney disease. The pressure often drops to normal with a permanent weight loss.

■ Trimming excess weight helps to increase the level of the HDL "good cholesterol" in the bloodstream, as explained in the chapter on cholesterol. Keeping weight down also helps a cholesterol-lowering diet work better, studies indicate.

■ A person's chances of developing diabetes double with every 20 percent over normal weight. And diabetics are twice as prone to heart disease as other people.

■ Losing weight can make a person more mobile, leading to a regular program of exercise that also may protect the heart, Daniel Halvorsen of the University of Minnesota's Laboratory of Physiological Hygiene noted.

But losing weight can be dangerous, too, if done wrong. To reduce safely, experts suggest never going on a diet of less than 1,200 calories a day — or taking off more than two pounds a week — without a doctor's approval.

What about fad diets?

Many are low-carbohydrate diets, which means the dieter consumes mostly the types of fats that raise the level of cholesterol in the blood, Halvorsen said. Higher cholesterol levels mean added heart risks. Some of these diets also make the people feel bad, because this isn't a normal way of eating.

"But my biggest concern is that they're not getting at the crux of the problem — they're not getting a permanent change in eating patterns," he said.

Calories to burn

The arithmetic of counting calories is important:

If you consume more calories than your body burns up, you gain weight. And vice versa.

For each 3,500 excess calories, you'll gain about one pound. This means that even 100 extra calories a day can add up to an extra pound of weight every five weeks. On the bright side, it means that (starting from a point where you aren't adding weight) cutting back about 500 calories a day will take off about a pound a week.

Your body burns some calories all the time. But the more physical activity you have, the more calories are burned. So it helps to add exercise to the equation.

A typical adult burns roughly 100 calories for each mile walked, jogged or run. (Surprised? Remember that you can jog a mile much more quickly than walk it, so if you're going to try to burn up a lot of calories walking would take more time. The work of moving the body a mile is essentially the same, regardless of how you do it, Halvorsen said.)

A discouraging way to think of it is:

1 pound of excess weight = 3,500 calories = 35 miles of jogging to take it off.

So think of it this way:

1 mile of extra walking a day (100 calories) x 365 days = 36,500 calories burned up = 10 pounds of weight in a year.

That's how adding a 20- to 30-minute stroll to your day can take pounds off your waistline — or, if you're already trim, help you stay that way.

What you can do:

On this list of suggestions from the Changing Weighs program at Metropolitan Medical Center, check the ones that can help you:

Time is on your side

Research has shown that regardless of how much you eat, it takes about 20 minutes from the first bite until the I've-had-enough satisfaction reaches your brain. So if you find yourself eating too much at meals or you are still hungry after a meal and craving a snack, here are some ways to slow down your eating:

☐ When you sit down, relax for a few seconds before starting to eat.

☐ Chew each mouthful of food slowly; don't pick up a second bite until you've completely chewed and swallowed the first.

☐ Put down your fork or spoon before picking up the next piece of food. And take a rest after eating several mouthfuls.

☐ Pay more attention to the taste and smell of your food.

☐ Begin each meal with a glass of water or iced tea.

☐ Select foods that require more work to eat, such as fish that hasn't been filleted or crab in the hard shell.

☐ Try to be the last person to finish each course of the meal.

Don't let feelings force you to the fridge

If you find you overeat when you're in a one mood or another, or when you feel a particular way, check the appropriate box and follow these tips:

☐ Do you overeat when you're tired? Take a nap or go to bed early when you get hungry. Or sit back and listen to music.

☐ Does tension trigger your overeating? Concentrate on muscle relaxation: Clench your fists and notice the tension in the muscles in your hands. Suddenly let your hands relax and enjoy the comfort you feel. You can do the same thing with the forearm muscles and other large muscle groups in your body.

☐ Do you turn to food when you're bored? Make a list of things that need to be done around the house, such as cleaning closets. Tackle these tasks the next time you feel hungry. This also may help reduce tension.

☐ Do you eat too much when feeling lonely? Phone someone. Or write a letter.

☐ Do you overeat when you're angry? Talk to someone who will be supportive. Or think about talking to the person you're angry with. Or hit a pillow. Or think pleasant thoughts, such as a vacation.

☐ Regardless of what mood triggers your eating, taking a walk may help overcome the urge to consume food. And it will *burn* some calories.

Beware of snacking

If snacking is your problem, select one or more tips out of this group:

☐ Do you overeat at lunch or crave goodies at a mid-morning break? Don't skip breakfast.

☐ Establish a rule that, while at home, you'll eat only while sitting in one particular place in the kitchen or dining room. You can have a snack, but it must be eaten there. Then you'll have to think about it when you eat. You won't be able to nibble away while watching TV but if you're really hungry, you can go to your designated eating spot.

☐ If you really want to snack, give yourself 10 minutes before you do. Your hunger may be psychological rather than physiological. Give it a chance to go away. But if you set this rule for yourself, you still know that you can get something to eat within 10 minutes anytime you're *really* hungry.

Avoid trips to temptation

Sometimes it's *where* you are that's the problem:

☐ If coffee breaks are your problem, take a Thermos with you so you don't have to go to the cafeteria or wherever you might be exposed to the rolls-and-coffee setting.

☐ Have a hard time passing the candy counter without stopping? Either try to avoid going past or tell yourself you'll eat only things you put on a list you write out.

☐ If you snack while preparing meals, try to fix them when you're not hungry. For example, prepare dinner immediately after eating lunch.

☐ Do you get an impulse to eat when you enter the front door of your home? Slow your pace by hanging up your coat and putting packages away. Or enter a door that won't take you though the kitchen. Or try some exercises. Or simply sit down and relax.

☐ Do you have trouble turning down food at parties? If the hostess tries to get you to eat food you haven't planned for, say, "No thanks." If your hostess replies, "Are you sure?" or "Just a little piece," don't back down. Say you're full. If you give in once, the hostess may never believe your first answer is your final decision.

☐ If you find you snack at a certain hour of the day, say 4 p.m., plan to get out of the home or office at that time of day. But avoid grocery shopping then.

☐ If your overeating occurs at restaurants, order first so you won't be influenced by other people's selections.

☐ If you overeat at movies or ball games, take low-calorie food with you.

☐ If you overeat when you serve food to guests, don't feel obliged to eat the food you serve your guests. You also can serve low-calorie foods and drinks, since your guests may be trying to keep pounds down too.

Tips for the cook

☐ If you snack while putting groceries away, ask a family member to put them away for you.

☐ If you eat while preparing a meal, clean up after preparing each dish. Start to soak and do the dirty dishes as they accumulate.

☐ When possible, prepare the next meal's casserole, meat loaf, etc., after completion of the previous meal — a time when you won't be hungry.

☐ After prepared food is served, refrigerate leftovers immediately.

☐ If you find you're combining eating with cleaning after a meal, brush your teeth after the meal to officially end it.

For you — and everyone

Some general tips:

☐ If you start consuming calories when you're thirsty, remember that water is the best thirst quencher.

☐ If you find yourself taking too large helpings at meals, try a smaller plate.

☐ After losing some weight, have your clothes altered. This makes it much easier for you to keep the pounds off than to put them back on.

Plan some activity

☐ Park your car several blocks from your destination and get in a little calorie-burning walking. You may save time, since you won't have to hunt for a parking place directly in front of where you're going.

☐ Take the stairs rather than the elevator. (You may want to set a two- or three-flight limit, at least to start.)

☐ If you're having company, plan some activity as well as food. Touch football isn't for everyone, but even a lawn game like croquet at least keeps you away from snack foods.

6/Exercise: Benefits and risks

Rep. Goodloe Byron, a 49-year-old Maryland congressman and veteran of six Boston Marathons, died of a heart attack after jogging 12 miles in what was to be a 15-mile outing.

Dying with him was the myth that marathoners are immune to fatal heart attacks.

With more and more people running the 26-mile marathon distance, the odds finally caught up with this unrealistic expectation for physical activity, said a panel of exercise experts at an American Heart Association scientific meeting.

Not that these doctors want to stifle the exercise boom. Anyone taking an early morning walk in downtown Dallas during the heart meeting had to dodge jogging physicians on the sidewalks.

But there's concern about exercise triggering heart attacks in susceptible individuals. So the heart association's experts advise:

Check with your doctor if you plan to start a strenuous exercise program. This is most important for anyone age 35 or older who has been leading a sedentary lifestyle.

It takes strenuous exercise to improve the efficiency of the heart — that is, to get the heart to pump more blood with less effort. This is called cardiovascular fitness or endurance.

While there's not yet proof that cardiovascular fitness also reduces the risk of heart attacks, there's growing evidence that it does.* And even more moderate physical activity probably helps cut the heart risk, at least indirectly.

Trying to pin down the protective role of exercise has been difficult.

Researchers in 1953 compared the heart attack rates of two groups of employees on London double-decker buses: the sedentary drivers versus the conductors who walked around collecting fares. The drivers had a significantly higher heart attack rate.

The problem with this and many similar studies is that self-selection factors can lead different people to take different jobs. Later studies showed that the London bus drivers, at the time they took their jobs, tended to be fatter and have higher blood pressures than the conductors. A person in vigorous good health may want an active job.

But a recent major study adds strong support to the theory that vigorous exercise, at least, really can reduce a person's risk of having a heart attack.

This study, of 17,000 Harvard alumni, found that those who regularly participated in strenuous physical activity such as jogging, swimming, tennis and mountain climbing had about a third fewer heart attacks than their inactive classmates.

When Dr. Ralph Pafenbarger looked at other heart risk factors among the Harvard men, he found that the protection of strenuous exercise was in large part independent of such things as smoking, overweight and cholesterol levels.

Still, questions have been raised about whether the healthier Harvard men might have been more inclined to take up strenuous exercise in the first place.

But Pafenbarger did find that alumni who had been varsity athletes as students were not protected against heart attacks in later life *unless* they continued a high level of physical activity. Conversely, men who weren't student athletes had a lower rate of attacks if they later took up strenuous exercise.

Dr. Jere Mitchell of the University of Texas' medical school in Dallas, head of the American Heart Association's committee on exercise, said four things are required to achieve the cardiovascular fitness sought to protect against heart attacks:

■ The exercise must be dynamic, not static. Weight lifting is static. What's needed is dynamic movement of large muscles, which means jogging, tennis, swimming, bike riding or any other activity that makes you move.

■ The exercise should raise your heart rate to between 70 and 85 percent of its maximum. The amount of exercise needed to do this varies from person to person, depending on condition and and other factors. Brisk walking may be strenuous enough for a some people who have been leading sedentary lives. (For how to calculate your "target zone," see the end of the chapter.)

■ The exercise should be done for 20 to 30 minutes at a time, keeping the heart rate in the target zone. Wind sprints — running very hard for only a minute or so — and other intense but brief periods of exercise don't help.

■ You probably have to exercise a minimum of three times a week to achieve the fitness desired; at least four times a week is preferable.

Because the idea is to put stress on the heart to improve its efficiency, there's a risk that this can trigger a heart attack in anyone whose coronary arteries already are narrowed by fatty deposits. That's the reason to check with a doctor before starting an exercise program — and then to take it up gradually.

Doctors often have such patients take a stress test. This means exercising by walking on a treadmill while an electrocardiogram (a reading of the electrical impulses that accompany each heartbeat) is taken to make sure that the heart works fine under this stress.

Such a test is expensive (typically about $100), and some experts believe it turns up too many "false positives." This means the test erroneously indicates that an individual shouldn't exercise, when there's really no risk.

So there's still plenty of controversy about exercise.

"If exercise was as preventive for coronary heart attacks as penicillin is for pneumonia, it would take about five cases to prove that it was that good. The fact that we are having to do all these studies with thousands of people (to find the value of exercise) shows it's not a cure-all," Mitchell said.

But while exercise isn't a wonder drug, he said, "I'm a great believer that it's important." While the direct benefits to the heart are debated, some of the indirect ways exercise may help are:

■ Strenuous exercise tends to raise the level of HDL "good" cholesterol in your blood. This unusual type of cholesterol, as explained in the chapter on cholesterol, appears to decrease your risk of heart attacks.

■ Any amount of exercise burns up calories, helping you to reduce or to keep in trim.

■ Once smokers start vigorous exercise, they often want to give up smoking. You don't see many joggers puffing away as they run.

■ Exercise — even an occasional walk around the block — often helps reduce tension.

What you can do:

Here are five things to keep in mind in designing your physical activity program:

Choose the right approach for *you*.

Select a type or types of physical activity that you will enjoy, since the aim is to make this a continuing part of your lifestyle.

The chart below compares different types of physical activity in an unusual — but very helpful — way. A typical adult burns 250 calories with these activities for the duration or distance listed:

Walking — cover 2.5 miles (100 calories per mile)
Jogging — cover 2.5 miles (same as walking, 100 calories per mile)
Bowling .... 1:00 hour
Cycling (slow) .... 1:10 hour
Cycling (fast) .... 0:35 hour
Croquet .... 1:45 hour
Dancing (slow step) .... 0:50 hour
Dancing (fast step) .... 0:30 hour
Fishing .... 1:50 hour
Gardening (leisure) .... 1:00 hour
Golfing (caddy) .... 1:00 hour
Golfing (carry clubs) .... 0:40 hour
Handball .... 0:25 hour
Horseback Riding .... 1:00 hour
Shuffleboard .... 1:15 hour
Skating (leisure) .... 0:45 hour
Skating (rapid) .... 0:25 hour
Skiing (cross-country) .... 0:15 hour

Skiing (downhill) .... 0:25 hour
Soccer .... 0:25 hour
Softball .... 0:45 hour
Swimming (leisure) .... 0:40 hour
Swimming (rapid) .... 0:20 hour
Tennis (singles) .... 0:45 hour
Tennis (doubles) .... 1:00 hour
Volleyball .... 1:00 hour

Figures in this chart, from the University of Minnesota's Laboratory of Physiological Hygiene, are averages. Caloric expenditure varies somewhat depending on your size. The more vigorous the activity, the quicker the calories will be expended.

Get your doctor's OK.

Make sure it's safe for you to do what you plan. Experts recommend a doctor's approval before starting a program of strenuous exercise.

Don't rush it.

Start your exercise program slowly and build up gradually over a few weeks or months.

Figure your target heart rate.

For maximium benefit to the heart, the level of exertion should be at a level that will condition the heart. This level falls between 70 and 85 percent of your maximal heart (or pulse) rate.

The doctor can tell you your maximal heart rate. Or you can figure a good approximation:

Subtract your age from 220. For example, if you're 40 years old and in normal health, your maximal heart rate would be about 180, and the pulse rate to aim for during exercise would be between 126 and 153 beats per minute.

Little heart conditioning occurs above or below this "target zone."

To determine whether you've reached your target zone, take your pulse while you exercise or immediately after exercise: Count the pulse beats for 10 seconds, then multiply by six.

Warm up — and cool down.

A 5- to 10-minute warmup period is recommended before starting exercise. Then, after 20 to 30 minutes of exercise in the target zone, there should be a 5- to 10-minute cooldown period during which you slowly reduce your level of physical activity rather than stopping abruptly.

7/Stress: Should you worry about it?

"It felt like there was somebody standing on my chest," recalled Richard Jacoves. "Then I passed out at my desk. I woke up in an oxygen tent in the hospital."

Jacoves was only 30 at the time. His coronary attack convinced him that he had to change his approach to life to save his life.

Until that fateful day in 1965, Jacoves said his life had been "work, work, work. I was a nervous wreck."

No longer, he said. "Superman exists only in the comics."

Jacoves, a New Orleans liquor wholesaler, is featured in a film produced by the Mental Health Association to show people how they can reduce their tensions, for better physical as well as mental health.

"In any business there is both challenge and anxiety," Jacoves said, "but I used to get more and more involved in my own stew."

Now whenever he feels tensions building up "I call time out," he said, forming a "T" with his hands like a quarterback calling for the referee to stop the clock. "I get away for a while, even if it's just to wash my hands and face."

Taking a break when stress builds up is one of 11 basic tips that the Mental Health Association offers for dealing with everyday tension.

But medical experts still debate how important stress may be in causing heart attacks. Even assuming that stress is important, there are questions about what types of stress or personality are most critical, and whether stress is so ingrained in a person's personality that it's impractical to try to get most people to change.

Two San Francisco cardiologists, Dr. Meyer Friedman and Dr. Ray Rosenman, have coined the term "Type A behavior" to describe the type of individual their research indicates is most vulnerable to a heart attack: aggressive, impatient, competitive and chronically rushing to get things done.

"Hurry sickness," they call it.

They studied 3,154 middle-aged men. Half were classified as having Type A behavior and the other half were found to be the easier-going Type B. Nine years later they found that 34 of the Type As but only 16 Type Bs had died of heart attacks. A similar increased risk also was found in the Type As for nonfatal coronary artery disease.

Critics say that a Type A person may be more likely to smoke, that the tensions in his life may contribute to high blood pressure, or that he may be a too-hearty eater (or snack nibbler) whose choices of foods force up his weight and cholesterol levels.

The Rosenman-Friedman study, however, concluded that this could explain only part of the increased heart risks they found among the Type A men. And while acknowledging that cholesterol levels tend to run higher among Type A people, they blame stress as a major reason rather than diet alone.

Because of such complicating factors, and the difficulty of classifying everyone neatly into either a Type A or Type B profile, the debate continues. Dr. Henry Blackburn of the University of Minnesota has raised some intriguing questions:

Why do the Japanese, known as one of the most competitive peoples in the world, who live a hustle-bustle life on that crowded island, have the lowest heart attack rate of any industrialized nation in the world?

Japanese who migrate to the United States develop American-style high coronary rates. Blackburn attributes this to the Japanese-Americans' picking up American eating habits. But, just to show how complicated things can get, University of California researchers blame American-style stress. So the debate continues.

Not that Blackburn dismisses the danger of stress. "There is no question that stress can be important," he said. "The question is *how*."

Blackburn said stress may be important for individuals who already have narrowed coronary arteries, caused by the buildup of cholesterol-rich deposits in the arteries that branch through the heart muscle. Here's how it might work:

Stress is known to affect the body's hormones, and also may affect the tiny platelets in the bloodstream that are involved in clotting. If a person already has narrowed coronary arteries, stress might play some contributing or triggering role in the final clot or spasm in a coronary artery that closes it.

When a coronary artery is closed, nourishing blood can't get through to a section of heart muscle. That's a heart attack.

So stress might not play an important role in triggering heart attacks among Japanese, whose low-fat diet keeps their coronary arteries from narrowing. But it might be important in the United States, where the high-fat diet has made narrowed coronary arteries much more common.

Stress "can be the precipitator of the final event," as Dr. Jeremiah Stamler of Northwestern University Medical School put it, and also may "add insult to injury" earlier in the process leading up to a heart attack.

Also, controlling stress may be very important in bringing other risk factors under control. Tension may be an important reason why a smoker can't give up cigarettes or a pudgy person can't stay away from snacks.

Don't think you have to change your job to get away from stress, however. You might find yourself in deeper water.

"The presidents of many banks and corporations — perhaps even the majority — may be Type B individuals," Friedman and Rosenman write in their best-selling book, "Type A Behavior and Your Heart." On the other hand, they say, janitors, shoe salesmen, truck drivers, architects and housewives may be Type As, depending on how they approach their jobs and lives.

Many Type B people "have drive, loads of it," but they "monitor it with a calendar, not a stopwatch," the San Francisco doctors say. The moral: You may get more accomplished in the long run if you don't get harried all the time rushing to meet self-imposed or other deadlines.

A Cornell University researcher spent seven years collecting data on

270,000 Bell System employees from coast to coast.

"The story didn't come out the way we expected," said Dr. Lawrence Hikle said in reporting the results about 10 years ago. The researchers found that the Bell Telephone executives had a much lower rate of disabling coronary heart disease (primarily heart attacks) than their company's workmen.

The annual rate, per thousand men aged 30 to 59, was 1.85 for the executives, 4.52 for foremen and 4.32 for workmen.

The effect of stress on the level of cholesterol in a person's blood also is intriguing.

Friedman and Rosenman followed the cholesterol levels of a group of accountants from January to June. The levels went up before the April 15 tax deadline, then fell in May and June.

Blackburn sought to put this in perspective, however.

"Stress is reponsible for acute fluctuations in cholesterol levels, but we aren't aware of any chronic (long-term) effects as yet," the University of Minnesota heart researcher said. And in all experiments in which long-term cholesterol levels have been linked to either personality types or stress, he said, diet has never been controlled.

So trying to sort all the factors is tricky.

Take Jacoves, who is convinced that bringing stress under control is the reason he hasn't had any further heart trouble.

"I'm a very lucky guy, super lucky," he said, noting that his coronary attack apparently was caused only by a temporary shutdown of a coronary artery that reopened before any lasting heart damage occurred.

Yes, he exercises more now, too. In fact, he now jogs. "It's relaxing for me," he said. "Running three miles is better than three martinis."

Yes, with stress reduced he doesn't eat snack foods as he once did, "and my cholesterol level is down."

So is it really the reduction in stress that has helped Jacoves? Or the other things? Or would the other changes to a more healthy lifestyle have occurred if he hadn't brought stress under control?

Whatever the case, stress is linked to a wide variety of other ills. It has been found to contribute to alcoholism, ulcers, headaches and mental illness. And it may leave a person run down and vulnerable to other ailments.

So you don't have to wait for all the answers about the complex way that stress may be linked to heart attacks before deciding to reduce the stress in your life. Relieving stress may save your life; it certainly will make your life more enjoyable.

What you can do:

Here's a quiz to see if your lifestyle fits into the Type A or Type B pattern that may influence your vulnerability to a heart attack:

Yes   No

☐   ☐   Do you hate waiting in line at the movies or restaurant?

☐   ☐   Do you always move, walk and eat fast?

☐   ☐   Do you frequently set deadlines for yourself?

☐   ☐   Do you often get irritated when the car in front of you slows down?

☐   ☐   Does it bother you watching a person do something you know you could do faster?

☐   ☐   Do you often try to do two things at once, like reading while you eat?

☐   ☐   Do you feel guilty when you relax and do nothing?

☐   ☐   Are you so competitive that you get upset when a child beats you at a game?

☐   ☐   Do you hurry the ends of your sentences — or skip them entirely?

Yes No
☐ ☐ Do you explosively accent key words in your sentences?

☐ ☐ Do you have aggressive or hostile feelings, especially toward competitive people?

If you answered yes to some of these questions, you may be falling into a Type A "hurry sickness" behavior pattern that has been linked to an increased risk of heart attacks.

If you're a Type A...

Here are suggestions on how to reduce the amount of Type A behavior in your life:

■ Eliminate unnecessary events and activities from your life.

■ Set aside plenty of time for each task you undertake.

■ Get up 15 minutes early to give yourself more time to dress and talk with your family without rushing.

■ Slow down your pace of eating, drinking, driving. Don't rush your life unnecessarily.

■ Find some time to read — or just to think.

■ Do one thing at a time.

"Remember that even Einstein, when tying his shoelaces, thought chiefly about the bow," Friedman and Rosenman write in their book, "Type A Behavior and Your Heart."

■ Remind yourself that speed and success are two different things.

"Tell yourself at least once a day," Friedman and Rosenman suggest, "that no enterprise ever failed because it was executed too slowly, too well."

To break everyday tension...

The Mental Health Association offers these 11 suggestions — to promote physical and mental health — for coping with everyday stresses:

■ Talk it out. Confide your worries to some level-headed person you can trust, whether a family member or someone else. This can relieve the strain on you, and discussing your problems may help you see what you can do about them.

■ Escape for a while. You can lose yourself in a movie, book, game — or maybe even a brief trip for a change of scene.

Making yourself "stand there and suffer" is a form of self-punishment, not a way to solve a problem.

■ Work off your anger. Pitch into some physical activity like gardening, cleaning out the garage, carpentry or some other do-it-yourself project.

■ Give in occasionally. If you yield, you often will find that other people will, too.

■ Do something for others. It will stop you from worrying about yourself.

■ Take one thing at a time. Take a few of the most urgent tasks and pitch into them, one at a time. Once you get these done, the rest will look relatively easy.

■ Shun the Superman urge. Don't expect to accomplish the impossible.

■ Go easy with your criticism. Instead of being critical about the other person's behavior, search out the good points and help him to develop them.

■ Give the other fellow a break. Tension often makes a person feel like he has to "get there first." It may be something as trivial as getting ahead on the highway. If enough people feel that way, everything becomes a race in which somebody will suffer, either physically or emotionally.

■ Make yourself available. If you feel left out, it may be because you've been shrinking away.

■ Schedule your recreation. Having definite hours for it will assure that you get in play to accompany your work.

8/Would you recognize a heart attack?

At first Kenneth Clark thought it was indigestion.

Then he thought he had the flu.

It wasn't until more than 24 hours after his symptoms began that Clark found out he was having a heart attack.

This Bloomington, Minn., man knows he's lucky to be alive.

"The confusion comes because most people have the mistaken impression that when you have a heart attack it's always going to knock you down and kill you," Clark said.

More than a million Americans suffer heart attacks each year, and more than 600,000 of them die. More that half of these deaths occur before the patient even reaches a hospital to take advantage of life-saving medical expertise.

Doctors say thousands of deaths could be prevented if everyone learned to recognize the symptoms of a possible heart attack, even though they vary some from case to case, and act quickly. Minutes often count.

Clark, a plumbing supply salesman, told his story:

The Clark family enjoyed a scrumptious noon meal on Sunday, Jan. 20, 1974. About an hour after he got up from the table, Clark, 48 at the time, had a burning feeling in his chest.

"It wasn't really what you would call pain, it was more just severe discomfort," he said.

Since he had never had heart trouble, he assumed he had eaten too much. Heartburn, he told himself, referring to indigestion in the esophagus or upper part of the stomach.

"It was a little high in the chest for heartburn, but that didn't register at the time," he said.

"I also felt quite weak. The symptoms continued for three or four hours. Then I took a nap. When I woke up most of the problem in the chest was gone, but I was still weak."

When he got up the next morning, his chest felt all right, "but I still felt washed out — very weak." He went to work anyway.

At noon he felt like eating only half a sandwich, then vomited. He started sweating a lot, and the weakness increased. The burning in the chest returned.

"And I looked pretty ashen, too."

He discarded the self-diagnosis of indigestion. Now he thought he had flu. At 1 p.m. he drove home, only about a mile from where he worked.

"I still wasn't thinking heart attack," he said.

About 4 o'clock he stuck a thermometer in his mouth and discovered he had no fever. Now doubting his diagnosis of flu, he picked up the phone to call his doctor. The physician, after a few questions, told Clark to get to the hospital. His wife drove him.

"I walked in, and the nurse bawled me out for that, but I didn't really think it was a heart attack." Tests quickly showed that it was. Minutes later, Clark was in the coronary care unit with electronic monitoring wires hooked to his chest and drugs flowing into his veins.

He spent 19 days in the hospital. Fortunately, he made an excellent recovery and hasn't had any problems since. But thinking back, he now knows that the delay in recognizing the symptoms of a developing heart attack could have cost him his life.

"A bomb with the fuse lit" is how Clark now refers to the time between his first symptoms and his arrival at the hospital.

Doctors define a full-fledged heart attack as one causing death to the patient or permanent damage to the heart muscle. Typically this occurs when a coronary artery is closed by a clot or spasm, shutting down the flow of blood to a section of heart muscle. Clark's doctor speculated that his coronary artery was only partly closed Sunday, then became fully closed Monday to make it a full-fledged heart attack.

So in some cases acting on symptoms early enough may catch a developing heart attack even before it has had a chance to cause lasting heart damage, heart experts note.

Delays in seeking medical help for heart attacks are surprisingly common. Studies show that heart attack patients delay an average of three hours from the time their symptoms appear until they call a doctor or hospital.

Why don't people recognize the symptoms? Experts offer three reasons:

■ "They expect something gigantic," said Dr. Brian Campion, chief of cardiology at St. Paul-Ramsey Medical Center. While some heart attack patients do collapse almost as soon as symptoms start, that doesn't happen in the large majority of cases.

■ It's human nature for people to want to deny that they are victims of something as serious as a heart attack. "It must be something else — I wouldn't be having a heart attack," they say. Or "It's probably not a heart attack — I don't want to embarrass myself by calling my doctor."

■ Heart attacks cause a variety of symptoms, in different combinations, which complicate knowing when an attack starts. Nevertheless, the American Heart Association began an effort several years ago to alert the public to the list of things that indicate a possible heart attack.

"Our first feeling was that this might make neurotics out of them," said Campion, past president of the Minnesota affiliate of the heart association. "But this hasn't been true. Doctors and hospital emergency rooms haven't been inundated with false alarms."

The severity of the chest pain or discomfort varies from one heart attack patient to another.

Clark said that while he didn't think about it at the time, not only was the chest discomfort a bit higher than usual for indigestion but also "I didn't have a bad taste in my mouth after vomiting."

However, Campion cautioned against expecting any specific thing to be a tipoff. "It doesn't have to be unusual," he said. Referring to the tendency for people to deny that they have had a heart attack, he said, "They make the unusual seem usual in their minds. Play it safe; it's no shame to be wrong."

He noted that the first few minutes after a heart attack are the most lethal, so any delay is dangerous.

"The majority of deaths occur within the first hour or so of symptoms," Campion said. "Once we get them into the medical care system, we can help."

What you should know:

The American Heart Association says you should know these symptoms of a possible heart attack:

■ Typically there is uncomfortable pressure, fullness, squeezing or pain in the center of the chest (behind the breastbone) lasting two minutes or more.

■ Pain may — but doesn't always — spread to the shoulders, arm, neck or jaw.

■ Severe pain, dizziness, fainting, sweating, nausea or shortness of breath may also occur. But again, these symptoms aren't always present.

■ Sometimes the symptoms subside, then return. Remember, they aren't always severe.

■ Momentary sharp, stabbing twinges of pain usually are not signals of a heart attack.

What to do:

■ Sit down or, if you feel faint, lie down.

■ If the symptoms last two minutes or longer, the heart association says, assume that it may be a heart attack until a professional medical person says otherwise.

■ If you are a friend or spouse of the person with the symptoms, don't be surprised by "denial"; it's common for a person to deny the possibility of anything as serious as a heart attack. Insist on taking prompt action. An American Heart Association slogan is: "Would you rather be embarrassed or dead?"

Whom to call

While many people will call their doctor first if the symptoms are vague, many heart experts now say that speed can be so important you should call an emergency medical service (rescue squad or ambulance) immediately.

In either case, you should have both numbers handy. Your doctor should be called second if you call the emergency service first.

Many experts also say it's often better to wait for the ambulance or rescue squad than to be driven to the hospital — unless you live in an area where there would be a lengthy wait. Trained emergency personnel can start helping as soon as they arrive. If the patient does go by car, somebody else should drive.

The inside cover of many telephone books lists the numbers for emergency medical service. It may be a police dispatcher, a fire department, a separate rescue squad or an ambulance service. If in doubt, check with your doctor's office.

[At the end of this book are cards listing the symptoms and other key information. They are perforated for removal, so that you can post them in your home, office or elsewhere.]

What to say

■ Give your precise address or location.

■ Say that a heart attack is suspected. If you're calling for someone who is unconscious and not moving, say a cardiac arrest is suspected.

9/CPR: First-aid for heart attacks

Frank Garrison of Edina, Minn., was bending over to putt on the 18th hole when he collapsed. He lay deadly still, a victim of cardiac arrest.

Members of the 56-year-old Garrison's foursome started trying to help, but none had any special training to aid a person whose heart had stopped beating.

Jim Hurley and Pat Haley, students at Edina-West High School, rushed from the nearby ninth green to take over. They were joined by Tom Beaver, a coach from Edina-East High School.

The students had been trained in cardio-pulmonary resuscitation (CPR). It's heart-attack first-aid: CPR can keep a person without a heartbeat alive until expert medical help arrives.

Quickly and efficiently the two students took turns pumping on Garrison's chest, 60 times each minute, to keep blood flowing to his brain. Mouth-to-mouth breathing by the coach supplied vital oxygen for Garrison's bloodstream.

The Edina Fire Department's paramedics arrived eight minutes after Garrison had keeled over. That's quick — but it wouldn't have been quick enough except for CPR. Without it, brain damage starts about four minutes after a person's heart stops beating. Death quickly follows.

The paramedics used an electrical paddle to shock Garrison's heart back into beating, then rushed him to the hospital.

"I feel wonderful now," Garrison said in a interview several months later, after he had returned to a fully active life. But he recalled how sore his chest felt for a while after the two young men had given him CPR.

"It's hard on your chest," he said with a laugh. "They have to knock the dickens out of you — but I'm very thankful."

Garrison, had suffered two very mild heart attacks several years before the golf course incident. But he had felt fine that April 1978 day until he got on the last hole and "began to feel a little woozy."

Garrison, who is in the home-moving business, is fully recovered now and continues to play golf.

Hurley, who has graduated from Edina-West, said of his role: "Anyone could do it — it's not hard if you've had the training. Knowing what to do comes back very quickly when you have to do it."

This is why the American Heart Association and other medical organizations are urging the public to learn CPR. Haley and Hurley learned it as part of their high-school health curriculum.

Here's what's involved in CPR:

The brain, the body's most sensitive organ, dies within a few minutes after the flow of oxygenated blood is cut off. That's why CPR must start quickly. The quicker it's started, the better the chance of survival.

CPR is taught in classes that typically take two or three hours. The instructors demonstrate how to make certain the patient's heart has really stopped (CPR can be dangerous otherwise) and how to do CPR alone or as a team.

The technique itself is as simple as ABC, with most of the class time used to get the feel of the technique by practicing on a life-size mannequin. In the alphabet of heart first-aid:

A is for airway. The first thing that must be done is to open the airway by tilting the head back.

B is for breathing, using mouth-to-mouth artificial respiration to puff air into the victim's lungs. Without this, there would be no oxygenated blood to pump, since the lungs stop when the heart stops.

C is for circulation. This means keeping blood circulating in the body — which is what keeps a person alive — by the 60 to 80 compressions a minute on the chest. Each push squeezes the heart and forces blood out into the body's network of arteries.

"To know how to achieve this, you really have to practice on a mannequin under the guidance of an instructor," said Dr. Patrick Lilja, chief of emergency medicine at North Memorial Medical Center in the Minneapolis area.

Because an untrained person could crack the rib of a "victim" who might only have fainted, doctors say CPR should be learned in a classroom rather than out of a book.

The word resuscitation may be misleading. CPR is not designed to revive the patient, although that occasionally happens. Just keeping blood flowing to the brain allows time for expert help to arrive, as in Garrison's case.

In most cities, while more and more people are learning CPR, the total number of people trained so far is still limited. So the number of successful cases in which CPR is started by laymen is still small.

And it's far from the perfect answer for heart attacks. Even if everyone were trained in CPR, many patients would die in their sleep or alone. And not everyone survives once he or she reaches a hospital.

But the more people trained in the CPR technique, the better the chances of success stories like Garrison's. That's being proven in Seattle, population 500,000, where one of every four residents has taken CPR courses.

Dr. Leonard Cobb, a leader in the Seattle program, said that each year more than 100 Seattle cardiac-arrest patients have CPR that's started by a layperson (before paramedics arrive) soon enough to have any chance of success. About 45 to 50 of these patients survive to leave the hospital. But Cobb said the CPR training deserves only part of the credit.

"One of the great misconceptions is that you can substitute this for an advanced emergency-care program," Cobb said. Trained emergency-service personnel must be able to respond quickly, taking over with their expertise and specialized equipment. CPR buys only time.

The few success stories like Garrison's in most cities so far, and even the larger number occurring in Seattle now, only dent the nation's heart toll of more than 600,000 deaths a year. That's why instruction in heart-attack prevention is also included in many CPR courses.

What you can do:

A growing number of organizations offer courses in cardio-pulmonary resuscitation (CPR). Here are five places you can check:

■ Your local American Heart Association affiliate.

■ The American Red Cross.

■ Your company's safety office.

■ The hospital in your community.

■ A rescue squad or, if the firemen in your community serve as paramedics, the fire department.

Cancer incidence by site and sex
Excluding non-melanoma skin cancer and carcinoma in situ (early cancerous changes) of uterine cervix.

Cancer deaths by site and sex

	Male			Female	
Skin	2% / 1%		Skin	2% / 1%	
Oral	5% / 3%		Oral	2% / 1%	
Lung	22% / 34%		Breast	27% / 19%	
Pancreas	3% / 5%		Lung	8% / 14%	
Colon & Rectum	14% / 12%		Pancreas	3% / 5%	
Prostate	17% / 10%		Colon & Rectum	15% / 15%	
Urinary	10% / 5%		Ovary	4% / 6%	
Leukemia & Lymphomas	8% / 9%		Uterus	13% / 6%	
All other	19% / 21%		Urinary	4% / 3%	
			All other	15% / 21%	
			Leukemia & Lymphomas	7% / 9%	

1979 estimated U. S. cancer deaths: 395,000
Total new cases diagnosed: about 750,000

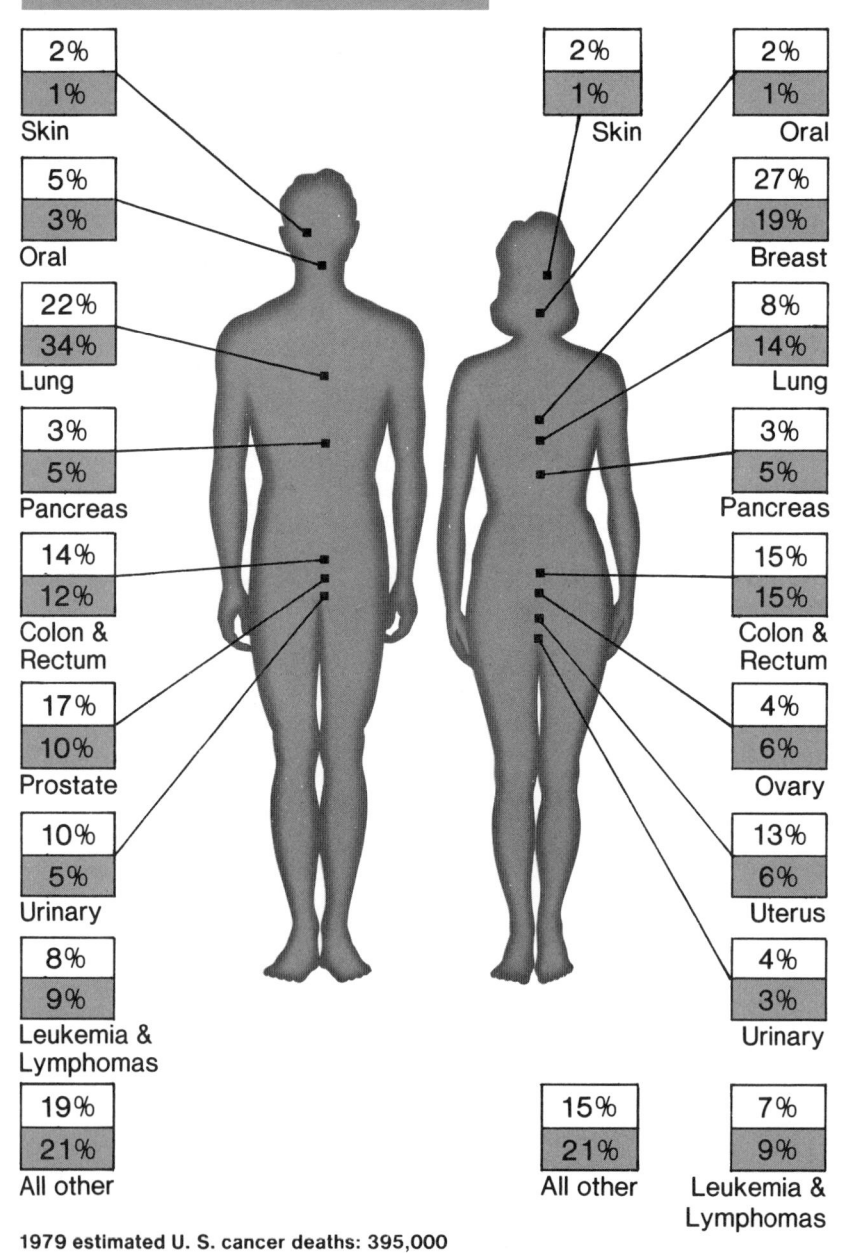

Cancer/
Cells that go berserk

There are trillions of microscopically-tiny cells in your body. In fact, the average adult has about 100 trillion cells.

That's 100,000,000,000,000 cells.

Cells are the ultra-tiny building blocks that make up all parts of the body, from bones to internal organs like the lungs and liver. Cells of different organs vary in shape and the jobs they do. But all cells reproduce themselves by dividing. This is part of normal growth and replacement of worn-out cells and repair of injured tissue. Thus cell division is essential to life itself — as long as it takes place in an orderly manner.

Cancer means that cells have gone berserk. Their division process has gone out of control. As the number of renegade cancer cells grows, building up into a tumor, they create havoc by overpowering normal cells.

When cancer cells spread through the bloodstream or the body's lymph (drainage) system, they can form the seeds of deadly new malignant tumors.

Cancer is actually more than 100 different diseases. For example, there are several different types of skin cancer, breast cancer, lung cancer, colon cancer, lymphoma (cancer of the lymph system) and others. Such complexity makes treatment of the disease extremely difficult.

For virtually all types of cancer, there are two lines of defense.

First, try to identify the many causes of cancer — and then do something about them. While medical researchers try to find more and more of these causes, much already is known. There'a a lot you can do to prevent cancer.

Second, if cancer hits you in spite of your efforts to prevent it, your chances of survival will be increased greatly if the cancer is found early. This allows surgery or radiation treatments to get rid of the cancer before it starts spreading.

10/Defusing the cancer time bomb

"I'd rather have a public that's scared than one that's not informed." —Dr. Frank Rauscher

"The quiet incubation period (of cancer) is probably responsible for the carefree initiation into cigarette smoking by adolescents." — Dr. Irving Selikoff

Your chances of having cancer depend, to a surprising extent, on the lifestyle you choose.

The continuing controversies over the the cancer-causing potential of everything from hair dyes to the artificial sweetener saccharin illustrate the growing scientific effort to pinpoint causes of cancer and do something about them.

But much can be done without waiting for more to be learned. Leading cancer experts say they already can tell Americans how to prevent more than 100,000 of the nation's annual cancer deaths. This represents more than a fourth of the nation's total cancer deaths, estimated at 395,000 a year now.

Cutting out cigarette smoking leads the list. Also on it are such steps as "prudent changes" in the American diet, curbing heavy drinking, cleaning up the workplace, using X-rays only when really necessary and having a healthy respect for the sun.

Most experts now agree that somewhere between 70 and 90 percent of all cancer cases have environmental causes. It's what we eat, drink, smoke, breathe or otherwise expose ourselves to that triggers the cancer.

It's scary. But hopeful, too. Identify the environmental factor. Do something about it. And you can prevent more cancer.

"We've only really begun to find these causes," said Dr. Irving Selikoff — a large, jolly, white-haired physician who heads the Environmental Sciences Laboratory at Mount Sinai Hospital in New York.

A growing number of animal tests and other evidence have linked certain food additives, drugs, chemicals and various other things — even sexual habits — to different types of cancer.

Early sex with multiple partners is associated with an increased risk of cervical cancer. Prostitutes, for example, are particularly vulnerable. While the reasons for this link between sexual activity and cervical cancer aren't clear, this association shows that cancer clues come from many directions.

Prevention: Weapon against cancer

Here's a look at some major ways for preventing cancer deaths:

■ An estimated 98,000 Americans a year die of lung cancer and experts say that about 80 to 85 percent of these cases are caused by cigarette smoking. That means about 80,000 lung cancer deaths each year are preventable. This alone makes smoking by far the leading known cause of cancer.

■ Heavy alcohol consumption has been shown to greatly increase the risk of a smoker's developing cancer of the esophagus (food pipe) and other areas in the throat and mouth. Alcohol apparently makes these areas of the body more vulnerable to the cancer-causing tars in cigarette smoke.

Overuse of alcohol combined with smoking accounts for about 5,000 more preventable deaths each year, said Dr. Marvin Schneiderman, associate director of the federal National Cancer Institute in Bethesda, Md.

■ There's good evidence, although not yet proof, that about 10,000 of the 42,000 annual deaths from cancer of the colon (large intestine) could be prevented by "prudent changes" in the American diet, Schneiderman said, and the breast cancer death toll might be lowered in the same way.

Prudent changes, he said, mean eating less animal fat, a step already recommended to decrease the risk of a heart attack, and at the same time eating more vegetables and fruits as a substitute. Countries with this type of diet have a lower incidence of these types of cancer, he noted.

■ An estimated 1,500 skin cancer deaths a year — a fourth of the total — could be prevented if people took reasonable steps to reduce repeated heavy overexposure to the sun, Schneiderman estimated. This may become more important "as our bathing suits get skimpier and skimpier, and we're out in the sun more and more with added leisure time," he said.

■ Many chemicals found in the workplace, from vinyl chloride used in the plastic industry to asbestos in the construction industry, are either known or suspected cancer-causing agents.

Schneiderman said that taking prudent protective steps, such as cleaning up the workplace and using available protective equipment, could reduce the cancer toll among industrial workers — without waiting for all the cancer-causing chemicals to be identified. He noted that clean water and good sewers virtually eliminated cholera in Europe before experts discovered the cholera germ.

It's difficult to separate the combined effects of cigarette smoking and industrial exposure in many kidney and bladder cancer cases. But Schneiderman estimated that about 5,000 industrially-related deaths of bladder, kidney and liver cancer could be prevented each year by reducing smoking and cleaning up the workplace.

Chapter 12 tells how X-rays and certain drugs can increase your cancer risks — and what you can do to reduce these risks. Chapter 13 explains prudent steps to take with chemicals in your home and in what you eat or drink. While precise estimates are difficult to make, thousands more lives potentially could be saved.

So while NOT smoking is clearly the No. 1 way of preventing cancer, it's far from the only approach. "There are a lot of things you can do for yourself," as Schneiderman put it — even though across the nation widespread changes in lifestyle aren't going to be accomplished overnight.

Schneiderman also noted there would be a time lag before many of the recommended actions would provide the full protection they offer. Studies indicate, for example, that it takes about two years after a person stops smoking before his or her lung cancer risks start falling appreciably — and about a decade to get the full health effect. Therefore, the best method of prevention is not to take up smoking in the first place.

Regulations may require cleanups

Other efforts to reduce the cancer toll will require regulatory action. In some cases, this means taking products with suspected cancer-causing chemicals off the market (such as was done with children's sleepwear treated with the suspect chemical Tris). In other cases, strict limits must be set on workers' on-the-job exposure to a cancer-causing substance (such as has been done with asbestos).

But again, you don't have to identify a specific chemical before taking prudent action. Some pollutants in the air and water that many Americans breathe and drink are suspected cancer-causing substances, so cleaning up the general environment may be another way of reducing the cancer toll.

Still, it's best to find the specific culprit whenever you can. So the continuing efforts to identify food additives, chemicals in the workplace and other environmental agents that may cause cancer are moving into high gear. The National Cancer Institute has long-term (typically three years) animal studies under way for about 200 other chemicals, and other tests are under way elsewhere. Federal law now requires more testing by industries that introduce new chemicals.

Learning from the Mormons

Many of the clues to preventing cancer, however, have come not out of the labs, but rather though the study of population groups. One of the most intriguing has been the study of 400,000 Mormons who live in California.

Dr. James E. Enstrom, a medical researcher at the University of California at Los Angeles, found that the cancer death rate among Mormons in his state is only about 55 percent as high as the average for all residents of California.

The rules of the Mormon Church call for no drinking or smoking, a healthy diet (particularly the use of wholesome grains and fruits, and limits on meat), no use of addictive drugs and, generally, moderation in life style.

Because of the no-smoking rule, the low incidence of lung cancer among Mormons isn't surprising. But Enstrom also found cancer-death-rate reductions of 30 percent or more for malignancies of the breast, colon, prostate, kidney, uterus and some other body sites.

Many countries have lower rates for various types of cancer than the United States. For example, there's much less colon cancer in Japan than in the United States, but when Japanese migrate to the United States and adopt American eating habits their chances of getting colon cancer increase.

So experts, by looking at different countries and the people who move from one to another, can figure out the lowest possible rates for various types of cancer.

It's on the basis of all this research that experts now believe 70 to 90 percent of all cancer is, one way or another, environmentally caused. Two unusual ways that environmental causes of cancer work should be kept in mind:

The "time bomb effect"

Although there are exceptions, most types of cancer don't appear until 20 years or longer after first exposure to the cancer-causing agent. Hence youngsters starting to smoke today don't have to worry about lung cancer — until they're in their 40s or 50s.

This lag provides time for preventive action: Stopping exposure to the cancer-causing substance, whether cigarette smoke or an industrial chemical or something else, greatly reduces any risk. But this time lag also may lull many people into taking a fatalistic approach.

"The quiet incubation period is probably responsible for the carefree initiation into cigarette smoking among adolescents," said Selikoff. It also means that a new chemical or food additive introduced into the environment today probably won't show its cancer potential for two or more decades — unless animal tests identify the threat.

The "chemical roulette" factor

Not everyone who smokes or is exposed to any cancer-causing substance develops cancer. Not every smoker gets lung cancer, for example.

Dosage, duration of exposure, genetic factors in the individual, the elements of chance — all appear to play a role in determining who gets cancer. No one can guarantee that you won't. But experts are now saying that there are prudent steps you can take to improve your chances.

Some experts still worry that all this talk about causes of cancer will cause "cancerphobia."

"I'd rather have a public scared than one that's not informed," said Dr. Frank Rauscher, former head of the National Cancer Institute and now senior vice president of the American Cancer Society. "I think the bottom line is that more Americans than ever before are aware of things and habits that aren't good for them. And that's good."

11/Smoking and cancer

Most smokers want to quit.

A Gallup survey for the American Cancer Society asked pack-a-day-or-heavier cigarette smokers: "If there was an easy way to stop smoking, would you do so or not?"

Two out of every three smokers — 67 percent — said they would stop.

While giving up smoking isn't always easy, there are a lot of ways to make it easier — and increase your chance for success.

If you are a smoker and want to give up cigarettes, here are four key steps:

Step 1: Consider your choices

Realize you do have a choice. Thirty million Americans have quit smoking.

Consider the payoffs of stopping:

■ It will greatly reduce your risk of developing not only lung cancer but several other types of malignancies — in addition to helping protect your heart and health in other ways.

■ It will save you money. Calculate how much you spend each year on cigarettes; add any costs you have from cigarette-caused damage to your clothes or furniture.

■ Quitting will get rid of the smell on your breath and clothes.

■ If there are teen-age or younger children in your home, ask yourself: Do you want them to pick up the smoking habit? "Parents who smoke are likely to have children who smoke, and teen-agers with two smoking parents are more than twice as likely to smoke as those with nonsmoking parents," according to a National Cancer Institute report.

■ Non-smokers are, more and more, speaking out about the annoyance and discomfort from cigarette smoke drifting or blown their way. No-smoking areas are appearing in a growing number of restaurants and other public places. It may be easier to quit than to keep smoking. Remember, the majority of American adults — 65 percent — don't smoke cigarettes.

■ "And quitting is taking control, being in charge of yourself," said Eileen Rotman, who runs an Unsmoke smoking-cessation program at several hospitals and clinics and also is on the faculty at the University of Minnesota School of Public Health.

After considering these and any other reasons you may have for quitting, list all the things you enjoy doing more than smoking. It may surprise you how many activities in your life you enjoy more.

Step 2: Just why do you smoke?

Find out *why* you smoke by using the quiz at the end of this chapter.

"There's no question about it, people use cigarettes in different ways," said Dr. Daniel Horn, a leading government smoking expert.

Is tension-reduction a major factor in your smoking? Habit? Simply the need to hold something? Other factors? The quiz shows you the reason or reasons you smoke — and then provides you with a tailor-made approach to quitting.

Step 3: Select your guiding choices

You have more choices. Plenty of them.

The National Cancer Institute has compiled a long list of tips that former smokers say helped them most to give up their habit.

On the basis of both the quiz and your own preferences, select the tips you think will help you from the long list at the end of this chapter.

Step 4: Watch for some good signs

Look for a couple of important benchmarks along the no-smoking road:

■ Within three or four weeks — sometimes sooner — most people start feeling better than they did when they smoked, Rotman said. Taste and smell improve. It's something to look forward to.

■ Then, "the first three months are critical" in dropping the habit, she said.

Giving up smoking is a lifetime commitment, but knowing these benchmarks along the way help you stick with your decision.

Your doctor's support will help

The Minneapolis Tribune's Minnesota Poll came up with a surprise finding in 1977: 60 percent of the smokers surveyed said their physicians had never suggested they quit.

Dr. John Witte, a smoking expert at the federal Center for Disease Control in Atlanta, Ga., commenting on the results at the time, called the lack of pressure by many physicians to get all their patients to stop "disturbing."

Dr. R. Lee Clark of the University of Texas Cancer Center in Houston, then president of the American Cancer Society, said he hoped doctors would begin speaking out to their smoker-patients because physicians are "the single most important factor in getting the people to comply on health matters."

It's not known if more doctors are speaking to their smoker-patients about the risk. In any case, if you plan to stop smoking, it may help you to bring up the subject with your doctor. He's sure to know that the medical evidence against smoking is staggering.

The bad news

An earlier chapter detailed the heart-attack risk.

Smoking is the leading single known cause of cancer. Experts note that smoking is responsible for at least 80 percent (many experts say 85 percent) of the lung cancer deaths. And lung cancer takes about 98,000 lives a year in the United States.

"I think many smokers don't appreciate that we are dealing with other cancer sites in addition to the lungs," said Dr. Arthur Upton, head of the National Cancer Institute.

Smokers have significantly higher rates of cancer of the larynx, throat, mouth and esophagus (food pipe). That's not surprising; all these sites are along routes that smoke can travel.

Cigarette smoking also increases the risk of kidney and bladder cancer. The reason: The kidneys extract waste products from the bloodstream, turning them into urine. These chemicals include tars from cigarette smoke, which get into the blood through the lungs. These tars and other cancer-causing chemicals become concentrated in the urine, which is stored in the bladder before it's expelled from the body.

Smoking also increases the risk of cancer of the pancreas, since that organ appears particularly sensitive to smoking-related chemicals that get into the bloodstream.

The good news

But there's good news: Stopping smoking does help. The risks drop until almost all danger of past smoking has ended 10 years after you quit. Of course that 10-year clock won't start ticking until you stop smoking.

While there are now 30 million Americans who are former smokers, there are 54 million who still smoke. Realistically, said Horn, eveyone isn't going to stop — even though the only fully safe cigarette is one that never gets lit.

So the federal government's anti-smoking program several years ago came up with five tips "to take *some* of the danger out of smoking."

These tips are based on studies showing that the more you smoke, the greater the risk. They also are based on research showing that reducing the tar and nicotine content of cigarettes reduces the risk of cancer and, to a lesser extent, heart disease.

For example, a study by Dr. E. Cuyler Hammond of the American Cancer Society found that smokers of low-tar cigarettes had a lung-cancer death rate 26 percent lower than smokers of more-potent cigarettes. However, non-smokers had a lung-cancer death rate *85 percent lower that even the low-tar smokers.*

This study was started before some of the very-low-tar cigarettes became widely available. But as the U.S. surgeon general, Dr. Julius Richmond, put it, "While some cigarettes are less hazardous than others," there "is no known safe level of smoking of any cigarette of any type."

So trying to make smoking safer is a compromise. With this in mind, here's how Horn described the five ways a smoker can cut his or her risks:

Tip 1: "Less glop"

"Use a cigarette with less glop — I don't know a better word for it," he said. That means less tar, which is the cancer culprit, and less nicotine, which affects the heart. But a word of caution: "Don't make such a big jump that there is a feeling of dissatisfaction. Go to a 20 to 30 percent lower tar first, then to lower and lower tar-content cigarette." (Rotman, as noted in Chapter 4, suggests changing brands each time you buy a full pack, until you're down to a very low tar brand in about five weeks.)

Tip 2: Smoke 'em just halfway down

Don't smoke your cigarettes all the way down. You get the most tar and nicotine from the last few puffs.

Tip 3: Don't make it a drag race

Take fewer draws on each cigarette and you'll be cutting down on smoking without really missing it.

Tip 4: Puff, don't always inhale

Reduce your inhaling. Don't inhale as deeply. Take short, shallow drags or just puff.

Tip 5: Deny yourself a few

Smoke fewer cigarettes each day. Select a time of day when you promise yourself not to smoke, such as at breakfast or on the way home from work. Think of it as postponing rather than cutting down.

Cut down, quit — or don't start

Horn said that while giving up cigarettes is by far the best approach, he wasn't worried that advice on reducing the hazards of smoking would encourage people to keep the habit. "Some find quitting too difficult," he said. "Cutting down makes it easier to quit later on."

A big concern is the new generation of smokers. The American Cancer Society conducted a survey of teen-age smokers to get some idea of what factors might induce youngsters to give up this habit.

For boys, the most important motives for not smoking were sports and physical fitness. Girls worried more about the health hazards of smoking, including the effect their smoking could have on their future offspring. Girls also worried more than boys about bad breath and cigarette odor.

What you can do:

Should a smoker quit "cold turkey" — or taper off cigarettes?

Why does one trick help your neighbor stop smoking but provide absolutely no help for you?

Research has shown that smokers use cigarettes for one or more of six reasons. This quiz, developed in the federal government's anti-smoking program, can help a smoker identify his or her own reason or reasons for using cigarettes — and then find a tailor-made way to stop.

After you take the following quiz, check the box — or boxes — that you score high or fairly high on:

Why do you smoke?

Here are some statements made by people to describe what they get out of smoking cigarettes. How often do you feel this way when smoking them? Circle one number for each statement.

Important: Answer every question.

	Always	Frequently	Occasionally	Seldom	Never
A. I smoke cigarettes in order to keep myself from slowing down.	5	4	3	2	1
B. Handling a cigarette is part of the enjoyment of smoking it.	5	4	3	2	1

	Always	Fre-quently	Occa-sionally	Seldom	Never
C. Smoking cigarettes is pleasant and relaxing.	5	4	3	2	1
D. I light up a cigarette when I feel angry about something.	5	4	3	2	1
E. When I have run out of cigarettes I find it almost unbearable until I can get them.	5	4	3	2	1
F. I smoke cigarettes automatically without even being aware of it.	5	4	3	2	1
G. I smoke cigarettes to stimulate me, to perk myself up.	5	4	3	2	1
H. Part of the enjoyment of smoking a cigarette comes from the steps I take to light up.	5	4	3	2	1
I. I find cigarettes pleasurable.	5	4	3	2	1
J. When I feel uncomfortable or upset about something, I light up a cigarette.	5	4	3	2	1
K. I am very much aware of the fact when I am not smoking a cigarette.	5	4	3	2	1
L. I light up a cigarette without realizing I still have one burning in the ashtray.	5	4	3	2	1
M. I smoke cigarettes to give me a "lift."	5	4	3	2	1
N. When I smoke a cigarette, part of the enjoyment is watching the smoke as I exhale it.	5	4	3	2	1
O. I want a cigarette most when I am comfortable and relaxed.	5	4	3	2	1
P. When I feel "blue" or want to take my mind off cares and worries, I smoke cigarettes.	5	4	3	2	1
Q. I get a real gnawing hunger for a cigarette when I haven't smoked for a while.	5	4	3	2	1
R. I've found a cigarette in my mouth and didn't remember putting it there.	5	4	3	2	1

How to score:

1. Enter the numbers you have circled to the test questions in the spaces below, putting the number you have circled to Question A over line A, to Question B over line B, etc.

2. Total the three scores on each line to get your totals. For example, the sum of your scores over lines A, G, and M gives you your score on Stimulation—lines B, H, and N give the score on Handling, etc.

Totals

___ + ___ + ___ = _____
A   G   M   Stimulation

___ + ___ + ___ = _____
B   H   N   Handling

___ + ___ + ___ = _____
C   I   O   Pleasurable Relaxation

___ + ___ + ___ = _____
D   J   P   Tension Reduction

___ + ___ + ___ = _____
E   K   Q   Craving: Psychological Addiction

___ + ___ + ___ = _____
F   L   R   Habit

Scores can vary from 3 to 15. Any score 11 and above is high; any score 7 and below is low.

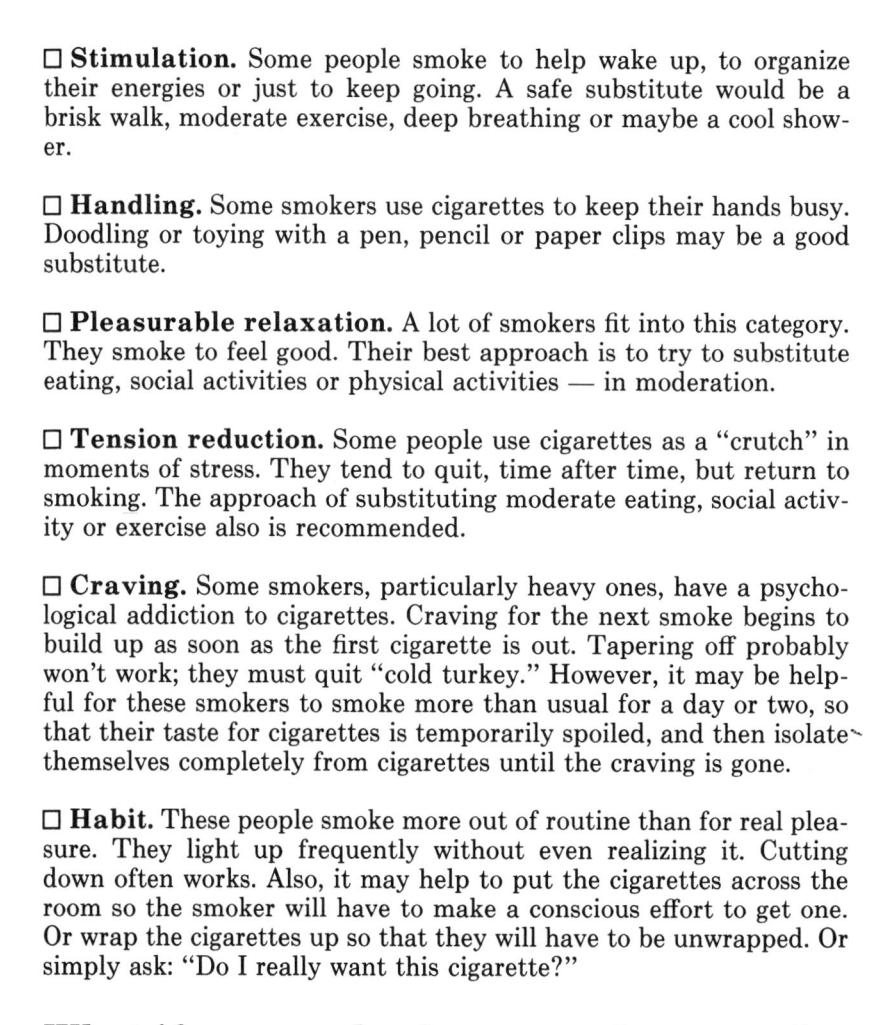

☐ **Stimulation.** Some people smoke to help wake up, to organize their energies or just to keep going. A safe substitute would be a brisk walk, moderate exercise, deep breathing or maybe a cool shower.

☐ **Handling.** Some smokers use cigarettes to keep their hands busy. Doodling or toying with a pen, pencil or paper clips may be a good substitute.

☐ **Pleasurable relaxation.** A lot of smokers fit into this category. They smoke to feel good. Their best approach is to try to substitute eating, social activities or physical activities — in moderation.

☐ **Tension reduction.** Some people use cigarettes as a "crutch" in moments of stress. They tend to quit, time after time, but return to smoking. The approach of substituting moderate eating, social activity or exercise also is recommended.

☐ **Craving.** Some smokers, particularly heavy ones, have a psychological addiction to cigarettes. Craving for the next smoke begins to build up as soon as the first cigarette is out. Tapering off probably won't work; they must quit "cold turkey." However, it may be helpful for these smokers to smoke more than usual for a day or two, so that their taste for cigarettes is temporarily spoiled, and then isolate themselves completely from cigarettes until the craving is gone.

☐ **Habit.** These people smoke more out of routine than for real pleasure. They light up frequently without even realizing it. Cutting down often works. Also, it may help to put the cigarettes across the room so the smoker will have to make a conscious effort to get one. Or wrap the cigarettes up so that they will have to be unwrapped. Or simply ask: "Do I really want this cigarette?"

What if you smoke for several reasons?

A smoker who scores high in several categories gets several kinds of satisfaction from smoking and will have to find a combination of solutions.

Those who score high on both craving and "crutch" use may have a particularly hard time quitting, but experts say it can be done. It's suggested they quit "cold turkey" — as recommended for craving-type smokers — but then they must be prepared for the craving to return at times. Or they may have to change their pattern of smoking (fewer cigarettes, smoked only halfway down and inhaled less deeply) first and then try the "cold turkey" approach.

If the quiz doesn't put you into either the taper-off or cold turkey category, Dr. Horn has a practical suggestion: "Throw your cigarettes away and, if it doesn't work, then taper off."

To help you stop smoking

The National Cancer Institute has prepared a list of suggestions that successful quitters say have most helped them give up cigarettes. Check the ones you think would help you — and use them:

When thinking about quitting

☐ List all the reasons why you want to quit. Every night before going to bed, repeat one of the reasons 10 times.

☐ Decide positively that you want to quit. Try to avoid negative thoughts about how difficult it might be.

☐ Develop strong personal reasons in addition to your health and obligations to others. For example, think of all the time you waste taking cigarette breaks, rushing out to buy a pack, hunting a light, etc.

☐ Set a target date for quitting — perhaps a special day like your birthday, your anniversary, a holiday. If you smoke heavily at work, quit during your vacation. Make the date sacred and don't let anything change it.

☐ Begin to condition yourself physically; start a modest exercise regimen. Drink more fluids. Get plenty of rest and avoid fatigue.

☐ Bet a friend you can quit on your target date. Put your cigarette money aside every day, and forfeit it if you smoke.

☐ Ask your spouse or a friend to quit with you.

☐ Switch to a brand you find distasteful.

Cut down on your smoking

If you want to cut down on smoking first, rather than quitting cold turkey:

☐ Smoke only half of each cigarette.

☐ Each day, postpone lighting your first cigarette one hour.

☐ Decide you will smoke only during odd or even hours of the day. (Smoke only from 1 to 2 o'clock, 3 to 4, 5 to 6, for instance. Or you might smoke from 2 to 3, 4 to 5, 6 to 7.)

☐ Decide beforehand how many cigarettes you'll smoke during the day. For each additional smoke, give a dollar to your favorite charity.

☐ Don't smoke when you first experience a craving. Wait several minutes. During this time, change your activity or talk to someone.

☐ Stop carrying cigarettes with you at home and at work. Make them difficult to get to.

☐ Smoke only under circumstances that are not especially pleasurable for you. If you like to smoke with others, smoke alone.

☐ Make yourself aware of each cigarette by using the opposite hand, or putting cigarettes in an unfamiliar location or different pocket to break the automatic reach.

☐ If you light up many times during the day without even thinking about it, try to look in a mirror each time you put a match to your cigarette — you may decide you don't need it.

☐ Don't smoke "automatically." Smoke only those you really want.

☐ Reach for a glass of juice instead of a cigarette for a "pick-me-up."

☐ Don't empty your ashtrays. This will remind you of how many cigarettes you have smoked each day, and the sight and smell of stale butts will be very unpleasant.

Just before quitting

☐ Smoke more heavily than usual so the experience becomes distasteful.

☐ Collect all your cigarette butts in one large glass container as a visual reminder of the filth smoking represents.

☐ Practice going without cigarettes. Don't think of never smoking again. Think of quitting in terms of one day at a time. Tell yourself you won't smoke today and then don't.

On the day you quit

☐ Throw away all cigarettes and matches. Hide lighters and ashtrays.

☐ Visit the dentist, and have your teeth cleaned to get rid of tobacco stains. Notice how nice they look and resolve to keep them that way.

☐ Make a list of things you'd like to buy yourself or someone else. Estimate the cost in terms of packs of cigarettes, and put the money aside to buy these presents.

☐ Keep very busy on the big day. Go to the movies, exercise, take long walks, go bike riding.

☐ Buy yourself a treat or do something special to celebrate.

Immediately after quitting

☐ The first few days after you quit, spend as much free time as possible in places where smoking is prohibited — libraries, museums, theaters, department stores, churches, etc.

☐ Drink large quantities of water and fruit juice.

☐ Try to avoid alcohol, coffee and other beverages with which you associate cigarette smoking.

☐ Strike up a conversation with someone instead of a match for a cigarette.

☐ If you miss the sensation of having a cigarette in your hand, play with something else — a pencil, a paper clip, a marble.

☐ If you miss having something in your mouth, try toothpicks or a fake cigarette.

Avoid temptation

☐ Instead of smoking after meals, get up from the table and brush your teeth or go for a walk.

☐ If you always smoke while driving, take public transportation for a while.

☐ Temporarily avoid situations you strongly associate with the pleasurable aspects of smoking — watching your favorite TV program, sitting in your favorite chair, having a cocktail before dinner, etc.

☐ Develop a clean, fresh, nonsmoking environment around yourself, at work and at home.

☐ Until you are confident of your ability to stay off cigarettes, limit your socializing to healthful, outdoor activities or situations where smoking is prohibited.

☐ If you must be in a situation where you'll be tempted to smoke (such as a cocktail or dinner party), try to associate with the nonsmokers there.

☐ Look at cigarette ads more critically to understand better the attempts to make individual brands appealing.

Find new habits

☐ Change your habits to make smoking difficult, impossible or unnecessary. Try activities such as swimming, jogging, tennis or handball. Wash your hands or the dishes when the desire for a cigarette is intense.

☐ Do things to maintain a clean mouth taste, such as brushing your teeth frequently, and using a mouthwash.

☐ Do things that require you to use your hands. Try crossword puzzles, needlework, gardening or household chores. Go bike riding; take the dog for a walk; give yourself a manicure; write letters; try new recipes.

☐ Stretch a lot.

☐ Get plenty of rest.

☐ Pay attention to your appearance. Look and feel sharp.

☐ Absorb yourself with activities that are the most meaningful, satisfying and important to you.

☐ Add more spontaneity and excitement to your daily routine.

When you get the "crazies"

☐ Keep oral substitutes on hand — things like carrots, pickles, sunflower seeds, apples, celery, raisins, sugarless gum and so on.

☐ Take 10 deep breaths, and hold the last one while lighting a match. Exhale slowly, and blow out the match. Pretend it's a cigarette and crush it out in an ashtray.

☐ Take a shower or bath if possible.

☐ Learn to relax quickly and deeply. Make yourself limp, visualize a soothing, pleasing situation and get away from it all for a moment. Concentrate on that peaceful image and nothing else.

☐ Light incense or a candle, instead of a cigarette.

☐ Never allow yourself to think that "one won't hurt" — it will.

Marking progress

☐ Each month, on the anniversary of your quit date, plan a special celebration.

☐ Periodically, write down new reasons why you are glad you quit, and post these reasons where you'll be sure to see them.

☐ Make up a calendar for the first 90 days. Cross off each day and indicate the money saved by not smoking.

☐ Set other intermediate target dates, and do something special with the money you've saved.

12/X-rays, drugs and cancer

As medical researchers spur their efforts to find the many causes of cancer, they're discovering some things to be concerned about in their own back yard.

X-rays and certain drugs can sometimes pose a risk of causing cancer. And identifying these risks is part of the effort to pinpoint the cancer dangers in our environment, then do something about them.

Some examples:

■ The National Cancer Institute has voiced concern about routine breast X-ray examinations in women under age 50 for the early detection of breast cancer. It's a sort of medical Catch 22. These X-rays can detect breast cancer at a very early, treatable stage — but the X-rays also may cause some breast cancer years later.

■ Relatively high-dose X-ray treatments were used commonly from the early 1920s through the 1950s to treat acne on the face, recurrent tonsillitis and some other problems in the head and the neck area. Now the National Cancer Institute is urging anyone who had such a treatment to check with his or her doctor. It's been shown that such treatments sometimes cause cancer of the thyroid gland in the neck from five to 35 or even more years after the X-rays.

■ Other warnings have been issued against general overuse of X-rays in medicine, since there's evidence that such radiation can cause leukemia and other types of cancer.

■ The Food and Drug Administration warns that studies show an increased risk of cancer of the uterus in women who use estrogen, a hormonal drug, for more than a year to treat menopause and postmenopause symptoms.

■ In the 1940s, 1950s and 1960s, an artificial hormone called DES was given to more than one million American women in an effort to prevent miscarriages. More than 200 cases of a rare type of vaginal and cervical cancer have been reported in the daughters of these women.

As potentially important as such findings are, some experts feel there has been overreaction by the public.

"Sadly, many American women have been frightened into believing that mammography (X-ray examination of the breasts) represents only danger, rather than a benefit," said Dr. Arthur Holleb, senior vice president of the American Cancer Society.

He expressed fear that many women who should have mammograms — because of their age, or a family history of breast cancer, or because they have symptoms such as a lump — will forgo needed exams because of their worry about the X-rays.

Mammography: When and why

The question of whether mammography actually can cause breast cancer still is not settled. But because very large doses of radiation (from A-bomb blasts in Japan and X-ray treatments for certain serious medical ailments) are known to increase the rate of breast cancer, most experts now think that smaller doses will cause breast cancer in at least some women.

Theoretically, a breast X-ray exam may raise a woman's risk of breast cancer by 1 percent, some experts calculate. Since the average American woman faces a 7 percent chance of developing breast cancer (it strikes about one out of every 14 women) in her lifetime, a single mammogram exam raises her risk to 7.07 percent.

So the National Cancer Institute says that mammography, except in a case where breast cancer already is suspected because of a lump or other symptom, should be used only when a woman's age or some other factor increases her risk of having breast cancer. Here's what the institute recommends:

"Because there is a small risk involved whenever a person is exposed to radiation, the National Cancer Institute believes that routine use of mammography for symptom-free women should be limited to:

■ "Women age 50 or over. Definite benefit from adding mammography to physical examination has been demonstrated in symptom-free women of this age group.

■ "Women age 35 through 49 who have had cancer in one breast. These women are at a risk about three times higher than average of developing cancer in the other breast.

■ "Women age 40 through 49 whose mother and/or sister (or sisters) have had breast cancer. These women are at a risk about two times higher than average of developing breast cancer.

"For women in these three categories, the benefits from routine mammography screening are believed to outweigh the small risks involved."

How often the mammography needs to be repeated varies by age and other factors.

Another tip: Before having a mammogram, a woman should ask her doctor how much radiation each breast will receive to make sure that modern equipment and techniques are being used.

"The dose per examination should not be more than one rad (a unit of radiation) per breast," says the National Cancer Institute.

Breast cancer is the leading cause of cancer deaths among American women, taking about 34,000 lives a year.

Three-quarters of all breast cancer cases occur after age 50. Monthly breast self-examinations and periodic manual examinations by a doctor can pick up many of the breast cancers than occur before that age — and are still considered "musts" even if mammography is used. X-rays still miss some breast cancer, and the monthly self-exam is the way to catch any breast lump that appears in the time between visits to a doctor.

Of course, regardless of a woman's age, an X-ray may be recommended by the doctor if a woman has a lump or other symptom of breast cancer.

Radiation and the thyroid

The extent of the thyroid-cancer risk posed by high-dose radiation treatments for ailments such as tonsillitis remains unclear.

The number of thyroid cancer cases has been increasing in recent years. One Chicago study of a thousand such radiation patients found 6 percent had developed thyroid cancer. Some other studies have reported similar rates. But at least two studies, including one at the Mayo Clinic, haven't turned up such a high rate, raising questions about different treatment dosages and how representative various study groups may be.

But at least 1 million Americans received such treatments, and some estimates run up to 4 million. Anyone who underwent such radiation treatments in the past should be checked by a doctor. Doctors usually can simply feel the neck to determine where there's any suspicious growth. Thyroid cancer tends to be a slow-growing tumor, so the survival rate is high unless the tumor is found late.

More about the National Cancer Institute's alerts for people exposed to this type of radiation, and for the daughters of women who received the drug DES in pregnancy, appears at the end of this chapter.

How about general diagnostic X-rays?

The number of cancer cases and deaths caused by other dental and medical X-rays is difficult to pin down. Doctors still debate how important a role X-rays may play in leukemia and some other types of cancer.

But the Food and Drug Administration estimated in 1976 that exposure to "avoidable radiation" — mostly medical X-rays — may cause as many as 1,800 cancer deaths a year in the United States. This includes the use of X-rays when they aren't clearly necessary, and the use of higher dosages of X-rays than are necessary with optimum techniques and equipment.

Some progress has been made in lowering the dosage of X-rays. But the basic concerns still exist.

Dr. Frank Rauscher of the American Cancer Society cautioned against any unnecessary X-ray exposure — including dental X-rays if they aren't really needed. "X-ray damage is cumulative," he said, "so even if your dose is very small you never lose it."

Dr. Arthur Upton, head of the National Cancer Institute, said: "I think the patient shouldn't have any, quote, 'routine,' unquote, X-rays. The guiding principle should be should be now that no (X-ray) film should be taken without some medical (or dental) reason." He said usually the physician or dentist can be the best judge of the need in a particular case, but "just to take a film as an annual routine, for example, without some medical reason is a mistake."

Upton noted that dental X-rays may reveal cavities between the teeth, but said "dentists today are encouraged not to routinely X-ray the teeth." He said that unless a person is prone to cavities, "taking a film every year isn't necessary and ought to be avoided."

He said there is probably no level of radiation exposure that's low enough to carry no risk at all. "This is the prevailing view today, and it represents a revolution in attitudes," he said. "Twenty years ago most observers would have argued that it took a fairly large dose. Today, I think, we accept that there's probably no threshold" below which radiation exposure carries no risk.

A list of suggestions to get the greatest benefit and the least risk out of medical and dental X-rays appears at the end of this chapter.

The estrogen problem

There was a 50 percent increase in the rate of cancer of the endometrium (lining of the uterus) among American women between 1969 and 1975, sounding an alarm that something was amiss.

Studies then showed a significantly increased risk of this type of cancer in women using estrogen for more than a year to treat menopausal symptoms. The risk was found greatest for the many women who continued to take the drug for many years in the elusive search for a "youthful forever" effect that some people claimed for it.

Women using estrogen after menopause appear to have a risk up to 10 times greater of developing cancer of the endometrium than women generally. It works out this way: A woman who doesn't take estrogen after menopause has about one chance in 1,000 each year of having this type of cancer. But a woman taking estrogen has 5 to 10 chances in 1,000 each year that she's taking the drug.

In all, about 37,000 cases of this type of cancer now occur each year.

The Food and Drug Administration says that there's a valid use for this drug in the short-term treatment of some women's menopausal symptoms such as hot flashes. But the agency still says that these women use estrogen only as long as necessary — and at the lowest dose that will control symptoms.

Doctors at first debated whether this risk was real. Some suggested that women who had undetected cancer might have symptoms making them more likely to use long-term estrogen therapy. But more and more studies leave little doubt that the there is a cause-and-effect relationship.

Now the good news. Dr. Marvin Schneiderman of the National Cancer Institute has cited dramatically encouraging evidence that things are turning around. In the first few years after this cancer risk received widespread attention in 1975, the sales of estrogen have fallen about 20 percent — and the incidence of endometrial cancer among American women has dropped almost 15 percent.

"This has important implications for both direct cancer prevention and for basic research in cancer induction," he said, "telling us that estrogens very likely are late-stage carcinogens or 'promoters,' and that the results of interfering with the action of a promoter can be seen in a very short time."

(The most common type of birth control pills contain estrogen along with another hormone, progestogen [progestin]. This combination apparently avoids the cancer risk of estrogen alone. Various cautions about using the Pill, including information on certain conditions that may indicate a woman shouldn't use the Pill, are listed in the patient-information sheet that comes with oral contraceptives.)

Experts also say that any women receiving menopause-type estrogen treatments should be particularly alert to any abnormal bleeding and have regular checkups by a doctor, so that any developing cancer can be caught at an early, treatable stage.

Other drugs: Only when needed

There have been some reports that ingredients in other drugs also may pose a cancer risk. As with X-rays, drugs — whether over-the-counter or prescription — should be used only when really needed. Cancer is just one of the risks that overuse of medications can pose.

But one caution: If you hear of any danger about a particular drug your doctor has told you to take, check first before you stop using it. Your doctor may prescribe a substitute — or tell you that the risk of not taking the drug is greater for you than taking it.

What you should know:

The National Cancer Institute has issued special alerts for two groups of people whose past medical treatments increase their risks of developing cancer:

■ The 1 million to 1.5 million American women who were exposed before birth to DES, a synthetic hormone. The drug was given to pregnant women to avoid threatened miscarriages.

■ At least 1 million Americans who, usually as children or young adults, had X-ray treatments involving the head or neck.

DES

Who: The daughters of any mothers who received a DES-type drug to prevent miscarriage. DES stands for diethylstilbestrol; it's sometimes just called stilbestrol. The drug was given primarily, but not exclusively, to women who had a history of problem pregnancies. It was used mostly from 1940 to 1970. Then it was discovered that the daughters of these women had an increased risk of developing clear-cell adenocarcinoma (an unusual type of cancer) of the vagina or cervix.

What to do: Daughters who might have been exposed before birth to DES or other DES-type drugs should be examined by a doctor if:

■ They have reached age 14, or earlier if they begin to menstruate before that age, or

■ They have abnormal signs such as bleeding or discharge from the vagina before their periods have begun.

"If possible, exposure to DES-type drugs before birth should be verified from medical records," says the National Cancer Institute. "But whether or not you are certain about exposure, play it safe and see a physician now." Annual checkups — or in some cases more frequent checkups if non-cancerous abnormalities are found — are then recommended.

The exam: It's fast, painless and can be done in a doctor's office. It's the standard Pap test with pelvic examination recommended for all adult women, plus a temporary staining of the vagina to enable the physician to see any abnormal areas. A magnifying instrument (colposcope) sometimes is used, too.

Most women in this group won't have any cancer. Even if a woman is found to have this type of malignancy, early treatment is highly effective.

The risk: A 1978 National Cancer Institute estimate of the cancer risk put it somewhere between one case in every 700 DES-exposed daughters, to one in every 7,000, based on what's known so far. Almost all cases reported so far have occurred between the ages of 14 and 24, with the peak occurrence at age 19. But it's too early to be sure that this will continue to be the pattern.

"We must keep in mind that these women (DES-exposed daughters) are still young," noted Dr. Upton, head of the National Cancer Institute. "We cannot yet be sure that DES exposure before birth may not adversely affect exposed daughters in later life."

(There has been one study indicating that there may be some increased risk of breast cancer in the mothers who took DES, but this isn't yet clear. Also, some studies have found an increased rate of some non-cancerous genital abnormalities in the sons of mothers who took DES, but so far this doesn't appear to be a major problem.)

Head and neck X-rays

Who: Anyone who, as a child or young adult, received X-ray *treatments* in the head or neck area. Typically, but not exclusively, such treatments were used for:

■ Ringworm of the scalp.

■ Enlargement of the thymus gland.

■ Deafness due to lymphoid tissue around the eustachian tubes.

■ Enlargments of the tonsils and adenoids.

■ Acne.

From the early 1920s through the 1950s, such radiation therapy was used extensively. Recent studies have shown that this can increase the risk of a person's developing thyroid cancer, since this gland in the neck frequently received some radiation during these treatments.

The alert does *not* include anyone who received dental or any other diagnostic X-rays, which use significantly lower doses of radiation.

What to do: If you think you might have had X-ray treatments in the head or neck area, don't delay. Contact a doctor and ask him to examine you. Then follow up with regular exams every one to two years. If you feel any growth in that area between checkup times, contact your doctor.

The exam: The doctor will feel the thyroid gland in your neck for any sign of a lump or swelling. The examination will take only a few minutes and isn't painful. Of course, if the doctor does detect some sign of trouble, more extensive tests may be needed.

The risk: The large majority of people exposed to such radiation don't develop tumors — and many thyroid tumors turn out to be noncancerous. (Even though at least a million Americans were exposed, thyroid cancer is still relatively uncommon, accounting for only 9,000 of the approximately 750,000 cancer cases diagnosed in the nation each year.) But this type of cancer can appear from five to more than 35 years after the radiation exposure.

Thyroid cancer doesn't spread quickly, so, if it is discovered early, it usually can be successfully removed.

X-ray guidelines

"As a radiation physicist, I wondered why my dentists took bite-wing X-rays of my whole family every six months. So I asked him how much radiation we were receiving. He became very, very angry. He said if I was planning to use that information to decide whether I was going to have a dental X-ray I could find another dentist."

This led Priscilla Laws, a physics professor at Dickinson College in Carlisle, Pa., to a new dentist — and to develop a Consumer's Guide to Avoiding Unnecessary Radiation Exposure. Some of her tips to reduce both the cancer and genetic risks of medical and dental X-rays:

■ Ask the doctor or dentist who proposes an X-ray exam to explain the benefit it will have for you. "Professional organizations, like the American College of Radiology and the American Medical and Dental Associations, have recommended that X-rays not be taken unless there are clear-cut clinical reasons to believe that they will contribute to a diagnosis," Laws says.

■ Ask if it's possible to use other recent X-rays instead of taking new ones. Too many doctors, she said, automatically say, "Why not shoot new ones?"

■ Express special concern about the need to X-ray children. Their cells are dividing as part of normal growth, and dividing cells are more susceptible to radiation effects. Also, children "have a longer remaining life expectancy, so that effects like leukemia and cancer have more time to manifest themselves in later years."

■ Tell your doctor if you think you may be pregnant, or even might become pregnant within three months. X-rays that expose a ripening egg, developing embryo or fetus should never be taken unless absolutely necessary, Laws says. X-rays of an unborn child can increase its chances of developing leukemia or other cancer in childhood.

■ When the X-ray machine operator says "Stay still," don't move a muscle. Movement can result in a blurred image and the need to retake the X-ray.

■ Question any dentist who insists on X-rays every time you have a checkup, unless you have many cavities or special problems.

■ Avoid use of the fluoroscope if your physician acknowledges that ordinary X-ray films will provide adequate information. Fluoroscopy is similar to taking an on-the-spot movie and it increases the radiation dose you get.

■ If you change doctors or dentist, or are referred to a specialist, have your X-rays transferred so new ones won't have to be taken. To make this easier, keep a list of X-rays you have received.

■ Question the need for routine pre-employment X-ray exams. Other tests may be given as a substitute, or previous X-rays may be used.

(The complete Laws guide, which contains extensive information about medical X-rays, is published by and available for $3.25 from the Health Research Group, Dept. 238, 2000 P St. NW, Suite 708, Washington, D.C., 20036.)

13/Chemicals, the sun and cancer

Is anything we eat or breathe safe any more?

Dr. Irving Selikoff of Mount Sinai Hospital in New York, who has dedicated his life to finding the causes of cancer, tells this story:

"In our hospital's corridors, a colleague will often stop to ask, only half in jest, 'Well, what's the carcinogen (cancer-causing agent) of the week?' The rejoinder suggests that the question almost answers itself: 'Is it better to know the causes of cancer, or not to know them?'"

More and more the headlines are filled with stories of new cancer risks. At times we seem to be swimming in a sea of carcinogens. And, in a way, we are. There's no escaping some exposure to a possible cancer-causing substance. Sunshine itself is everywhere — and its ultraviolet rays, in too high doses, can cause skin cancer.

Is it futile to try to fight such widespread threats? Absolutely not, the experts insist — because most chemicals do *not* cause cancer.

This chapter won't list every chemical that has been indicted as a possible cause of cancer. At its end, however, is a list of prudent steps you can take on the job, at home and at other times — including when you're out in the sun — to reduce your risk of getting cancer.

Can animals really represent us?

Public misunderstanding and controversy have surrounded a major research method used to find the causes of cancer: Using animals as stand-ins for people. How can scientists reach conclusions concerning human beings with tests involving a relatively small number of animals — especially when they're fed very large doses of the chemical being tested?

"I think a lot of myths have grown up about animal testing," said Dr. David P. Rall, a U.S. assistant surgeon general and director of the National Institute of Environmental Health Sciences at Research Triangle, N.C.

The biggest dispute has been over the efforts of federal health officials, so far stymied by Congress and the bureaucratic process, to ban or sharply limit use of the artificial sweetener saccharin. The Food and Drug Administration first proposed the action in 1977 after rats that were fed saccharin developed bladder cancer. The soft-drink industry — and many weight-conscious Americans — belittled that research.

If human beings had been fed the equivalent saccharin, the critics said, they would have had to drink 800 bottles of saccharin-sweetened diet pop a day for much of their lives.

It's time to demolish three commonly held myths about animal testing:

Myth: Feeding large amounts of anything to animals will cause cancer.

Fact: Experts say that most chemicals do not cause cancer when tested in animals — even though many chemicals have been chosen for testing because of their similarities to known cancer-causing agents.

The National Cancer Institute says that of the more than 7,000 chemicals tested throughout the world, only about 400 have been shown to definitely cause cancer in animals and 600 more have been found somewhat suspect.

Dr. Donald Kennedy, while commissioner of the Food and Drug Administration, said, "As a result of experimenting with thousands of substances, we have learned that too much of any substance will kill experimental animals. But only a small number of substances will cause cancer — in any amount."

Myth: The only fair test is to use smaller doses, more in keeping with human exposure.

Fact: The high-dosage testing is not only based on sound scientific principle, but it's the only practical approach available. Any food additive or other substance that causes cancer in even one out of 10,000 people could cause thousands of deaths in a nation the size of the United States.

But testing a chemical in several hundred animals, as is normally done, costs $500,000. It's expensive to allow mice to live out their 2½-year lifetimes under carefully controlled laboratory conditions and then to do all the microscopic and other scientific studies required to find any traces of cancer.

Because trying to test each chemical in more than a few hundred animals would be too expensive, the tests are conducted with large doses on a relatively small number of animals. If, for example, high-dose animal tests show that a substance causes cancer in 10 out of 100 animals, then at a very low dose it may cause cancer in roughly one out of every 10,000 human beings.

This is much more than guesswork. First, human experience shows that dosage does affect the degree of risk: A larger percentage of heavy smokers get lung cancer, for example, than light smokers. Also, where industrial exposure to a particular chemical has been proven to cause cancer, findings from animal experiments turn out to be a good index of risks.

Kennedy noted that there is a theory — of "which the chemical industry is understandably fond" — that there may be no risk at very low concentrations of a substance. But he said this "threshold hypothesis, apart from its suspicious convenience, should certainly be rejected on the grounds that no threshold has ever been detected for a carcinogen."

Myth: Rats and mice aren't anything like people.

Fact: The enzyme systems of these rodents are surprisingly similar to those of human beings. And, most significantly, among the 30-odd chemicals that have clearly been demonstrated to cause human cancer, all but one (arsenic) causes cancer in animals.

Because there are so many causes of cancer, it's very difficult to prove that any single chemical is responsible for even part of the human cancer problem. It took many years of research to prove that cigarette smoking causes cancer.

Most experts agree that saccharin isn't a particularly potent cause of cancer. But some estimate that it may cause 500 to 1,000 cases of bladder cancer annually among the many, many millions of Americans who use it.

A case can be advanced, however, for exempting calorie-free saccharin from the effort to remove as many cancer-causing substances as possible from the environment. After all, excess calories, avoided through use of saccharin, are a problem for many Americans. (See Chapter 5.)

But it's not that simple. Despite the widespread use of saccharin, the American epidemic of middle-age bulge has hardly vanished. Most people use the calories saved by saccharin to enjoy eating other things. It doesn't help to "save" 100 calories by drinking a diet pop — and then add add a 250-calorie dessert to your next meal. The potential benefits of saccharin often vanish more quickly than the pounds they are supposed to save.

Obviously, testing chemicals in human beings would provide more definite evidence that a chemical does cause cancer. But, equally obviously, there would be no volunteers. Ethics alone rule out such tests. So mice, rats and other laboratory animals are your stand-ins to find the causes of cancer. They get cancer so that you won't have to.

It was on the basis of animal tests, for example, that the flame-retardant chemical Tris, widely used in children's sleepware, was banned in 1977. But even before tests in animals showed this chemical had strong cancer-causing action, tests in bacteria pointed toward the same thing.

The Ames bacteria test, named for its developer, Dr. Bruce N. Ames of the University of California at Berkeley, can be completed in a few days rather than the several years animal tests take. The bacteria test looks for chemical-caused mutations (changes) in the bacteria's genetic material, which is believed to be a key way by which chemicals cause cancer.

The Ames test isn't considered nearly as accurate as animal tests. There is still controversy over it, in large part because many variations of the test have popped up across the country. It doesn't work all the time. But it can sound an alarm, as in the Tris case, leading to animal experiments. And it also may be useful for firms developing new chemicals to steer them away from substances that would pose future cancer dangers.

So test results of one type or another are coming "fast and furious now, because there's been a lot of testing in the last few years while there was very little before," said Dr. Sidney Wolfe, head of the Health Research Group that is part of Ralph Nader's consumer organization.

Some tests have found, and more will be finding, risks in consumer products. Other tests are continuing to identify risks in the workplace. Selikoff said this means Americans must be prepared to act on the findings.

If such knowledge isn't used to cut cancer risks, he said, "we would be, in a sense, biological bookkeepers," counting the cancer cases and deaths that might have been prevented.

What you should know:

The air you breathe, some of the foods you eat, the dye you use on your hair, the chemicals you use in your garden, the cleaners you use in your home, even the sunshine you enjoy — all can carry cancer risks.

But if you are aware of these risks, you can go a long way toward reducing your chances of getting cancer. There are prudent steps you can take at work and at home. Read about them, use them, for your own protection.

Chemicals where you work

The growing evidence that chemicals in our environment are a major cause of cancer was brought home when National Cancer Institute researchers compiled an atlas showing death rates from various types of cancer in each county across the nation.

The maps showed that areas where the chemical industry is concentrated tend to have high cancer rates. And the atlas pointed up the fact you don't have to identify each cancer-causing chemical before taking some action.

For example, the maps spurred efforts in New Jersey, where many counties showed up as "hot spots" for cancer, to launch a major cleanup of that state's big chemical industry.

Dr. Frank Rauscher of the American Cancer Society said this growing awareness of industrial-related cancer shows the need for more extensive and faithful use of existing protective equipment such as gloves, masks and respirators for industrial workers exposed to large amounts of chemicals.

"I know it's hot and sweaty to wear gloves," he said. However, because many chemicals haven't been tested for their cancer-causing potential, it's wise to reduce the amount of on-the-job exposure to chemicals in general. Studies clearly show that the greater the exposure to any carcinogen, the greater the risk.

Selikoff, of New York's Mount Sinai Hospital, said efforts are needed to educate workers about the value of such protective equipment. "Never overestimate a worker's knowledge or underestimate his intelligence," he said.

Asbestos — in many places

Asbestos is a needle-like mineral. Its ultra-tiny fibers apparently damage cells by puncturing or irritating them, rather than through direct chemical action. (This may open the way for chemicals, such as those those in cigarette smoke, to get into cells.)

Thus asbestos is different from most other cancer-causing agents. But it's a very important one that's just beginning to be understood. You can expect to hear more and more about this valuable but potentially dangerous substance.

Asbestos poses a special risk *both* on the job and at home.

Asbestos workers are known to have very high rates of lung cancer. Asbestos also can cause an unusual type of cancer called mesothelioma, which strikes the lining of the chest or abdomen. Asbestos workers also have above-average rates of cancer of the digestive system — esophagus, stomach, colon and rectum. And it's assumed, as with any cancer-causing substance, that exposure to a lesser, non-occupational amount of asbestos fibers still carries at least some risk.

Yet asbestos is common in everyday life. It's in brakelining and building materials and many, many other things. In fact, about 800,000 *tons* of asbestos are used in the United States each year. Asbestos has about 3,000 different uses, with about two-thirds of them in the construction industry for materials like insulation and floor and ceiling tiles.

As long as the asbestos stays in its intended form — such as in a piece of tile or other tightly bound contruction material — there's no risk, said Dr. E. Cuyler Hammond, a leading expert on the health effects of asbestos. The risk comes, he explained, when asbestos fibers are set free, creating asbestos dust that may be inhaled. Hammond, a vice president of the American Cancer Society, has done many of the pioneering asbestos-cancer studies in collaboration with Selikoff of Mount Sinai Hospital's Environmental Sciences Laboratory.

Asbestos at home — Some prudent precautions are recommended if you come into contact with asbestos during do-it-yourself home remodeling work.

"Unlike a gas or vapor, asbestos comes in clouds," Hammond said. "If you happen to inhale it, you may get more in one inhalation than somebody else might get in two weeks of it. Now if you have some asbestos insulation on, say, some old steam pipes in the basement, when this is ripped off you can get a cloud of dust. If you're going to do it, use a mask—and turn your head a little bit. A lot of these things are just common sense."

Asbestos consumer products — In 1977 the U.S. Consumer Product Safety Commission banned two products — consumer wall-patching compounds containing asbestos and artificial fireplace ash containing the mineral.

In 1979 the commission started investigating some brands of hand-held hair dryers that contained asbestos to see if they posed a hazard. Without waiting for the results of the study, some manufacturers offered replacements or repairs to eliminate the asbestos.

Your job — Now and even decades ago, a surprisingly large number of Americans have had occupational exposure to asbestos — and this has health officials concerned.

An estimated 1.5 million to 2.5 full-time or part-time Americans workers are exposed to significant amounts of asbestos dust in the construction and building trades, automotive brake and clutch installation and repair work, and the manufacture of a wide variety of asbestos products.

(While not every construction worker is at risk, many are. A worker usually knows if he or she is exposed to asbestos fibers that get into the air when the material is sawed, sprayed or handled in any way that releases the dust-like particles into the air.)

More than 4 million Americans worked in shipyards during World War II, when asbestos was used extensively in that industry. Therefore, many millions of Americans have had, at some period or another in their lives, occupational exposure to enough asbestos dust to pose a health concern.

Here's what the National Cancer Institute recommends for anyone who has current or past — even decades ago — occupational exposure to asbestos dust:

■ If you don't smoke, don't start. If you do, quit. While this is good advice for everyone, it's exceedingly important to people exposed to occupational levels of asbestos dust.

"Although asbestos exposure by itself can increase the risk of lung cancer to some degree, asbestos and cigarette smoking together increase the risk five-fold over the already high risk due to smoking alone," says a National Cancer Institute report. Quitting smoking is believed to greatly reduce — although not eliminate — this risk in asbestos workers.

■ Let your doctor know about your previous or current occupational asbestos exposure so he will be alert to any of the illnesses this may cause; this includes a lung condition called asbestosis as well as cancer. And have periodic checkups.

■ The federal government began to regulate asbestos exposure in the workplace in the late 1960s and this is expected to significantly reduce the risk. But anyone still working with asbestos should be sure take the recommended protective steps, such as using respirators for certain types of jobs and taking other steps to limit the amount of dust, to keep on-the-job exposure as low as possible.

In the water — Asbestos particles, which can come from either manufacturing processes or from the soil, have been found in some cities' water supplies. Researchers are trying to find out what the risks of ingesting asbestos fibers might be. Animal tests, along with studies of communities with asbestos in their water supply, are under way.

The sun: Too much is dangerous

"We have become a nation of sunworshipers," warns the American Cancer Society, pointing out that most of the 300,000 cases of skin cancer in the United States each year are caused by overexposure to the sun's ultraviolet rays.

While the risk of skin cancer is greatest in the Sunbelt states, many residents of the northern part of the United States also get this type of cancer. Fair-skinned people and those whose jobs keep them outdoors are particularly vulnerable.

Sunburn and prematurely aging skin also are problems with over-exposure to the sun. A single case of sunburn doesn't mean cancer, of course, but overexposure over the years does increase the risk. Here are some skin-saving tips from the cancer society:

■ Sun yourself before 10 a.m. and after 3 p.m., when ultraviolet rays are weakest. If that's too restrictive for you, limit your exposure at other times.

■ Remember that you're not fully protected in the shade of a beach umbrella. Ultraviolet rays are only partially deflected by the umbrella and they're bouncing toward you from all directions — off sand, water or the patio floor.

■ Don't count on being safe on a cloudy day or even under water. At least 70 percent of the ultraviolet rays' burning power penetrates clouds. The rays can even search you out three feet under water. A wet T-shirt also can deceive you, since water droplets funnel at least half of the ultraviolet power to your skin.

■ "The best cover-up available is a chemical one — any of the popular brand sunscreens that contain PABA," says the cancer society. PABA stands for para-amino-benzoic acid, which absorbs many ultraviolet rays but allows gradual tanning.

Most skin cancer is highly curable — unless it's found late or left untreated. An exception is a relatively uncommon but often deadly type called melanoma. Skin cancer, except for melanoma, is not included in the cancer society's estimate of about 750,000 cases a year of all types of life-threatening cancer in this country. Still, when regular skin cancer is found late or left untreated, serious scars and sometimes death can result.

Early warning signs for skin cancer include a sore that doesn't heal, change in the size or color of a wart or mole, or development of any unusual pigmented areas.

In and around your home

Pesticides, fungicides and other garden or lawn chemicals.
A number of pesticides have been shown to have cancer-causing potential, so this class of chemicals is suspect.

This doesn't mean all these chemicals cause cancer; they don't. It doesn't mean you shouldn't use them on your yard. What it means is that you should exercise care in their use, said Dr. Arthur Upton, head of the National Cancer Institute.

So follow instructions on the labels. Don't get these chemicals all over you when you use them. Keep the dust level down. Keep the chemicals away from children and their toys (youngsters put a lot of things they play with in their mouths). Store them in a safe place — and away from food.

Household solvent cleaners, cleaning fluids and paint thinners — The chemicals used in some of these products have been shown to cause cancer in animals, and thus presumably can do so in humans.

"I would use them prudently," Upton said. "I wouldn't go down in the basement with all the widows closed and just slosh the stuff around and inhale a concentrated atmosphere. I would not want to work in high concentrations over a long period of time."

When you eat

Some food dyes have been banned because of cancer risks. But one of the latest food additives to get attention is nitrites, commonly used as meat-curing preservatives in foods such as hams, bacon, hot dogs and some canned meats. Nitrites kill the germs that can cause deadly botulism. However, recent tests have show that this chemical can cause cancer in animals — and thus should be considered a cancer risk in man.

A growing number of experts are suggesting that the amounts of nitrites in these foods be cut back while a safe substitute is sought. In the meantime, you'll have to make your own decision about how much of these foods you want to eat.

Even charcoal broiling of food creates a small amount of a chemical that has been shown to have a cancer-causing capability. It's a benzo(a)pyrene, one of the many components in tobacco smoke, that is created with the charring of the barbecued food.

Researchers at Washington University in St. Louis, Mo., tested chemicals on bacteria — rather than animals — to measure genetic changes as an indication of cancer-causing capability. In the course of the tests they found, to their surprise, that something in fried hamburger meat might pose a slight cancer risk. When the hamburger was cooked in a broiler or microwave oven, the cancer-suspect substance wasn't produced.

Of course, tests with bacteria aren't considered nearly as reliable as tests using animals. But all this research has sparked new interest in studying safer ways of cooking food. The answers aren't in yet. "The degree to which they pose a cancer risk is still quite uncertain," the National Cancer Institute's Upton emphasized. "I wouldn't shun barbecued steak or hamburger — but I would think one would want to eat such food in moderation."

Many heart experts, for all the reasons detailed in Chapter 2, heartily agree.

Atop your head — and much higher

Thirty-five million American women — and an unknown number of men — use hair dyes.

Since a finding in 1977 that many permanent hair dyes contain chemicals that cause cancer when fed to rats, many of the companies that make hair-coloring products have been quietly removing the suspect chemicals and substituting others assumed to be safe.

The Food and Drug Administration has proposed — but not yet finally adopted — a regulation that would warn consumers of this finding. According to the proposal, dyes containing the suspect chemicals would carry a label saying: "Warning: Contains an ingredient that can penetrate your skin and has been determined to cause cancer in laboratory animals."

The hair-coloring industry has questioned the existence of any risk. Its officials have cited evidence ranging from how infrequently dyes are applied, to lack of evidence of an increased rate of cancer among beauticians who work with the dyes.

Meanwhile, you can look at the list of ingredients on the hair-dye box to see whether a product contains the suspect chemicals: 4-methoxy-m-phenylenediamine (4MMPD) and its sulfate (4MMPD sulfate). These chemicals also are known as 2,4 diaminoanisole (2, 4 DAA) and 2,4 DAA sulfate.

Another chemical cancer risk has been eliminated.

After years of concern, a government ban on virtually all aerosol products containing fluorocarbons went into effect in April 1979, following a two-year phaseout. Fluorocarbon propellants had been used to provide pressure for more than a billion containers of consumer products each year. But there was evidence that they damaged the upper atmosphere's ozone layer, which filters out some of the powerful ultraviolet rays that can cause skin cancer.

14/Your diet and cancer

You may be able to lower your risk of developing cancer by following the same prudent diet recommended in this book to protect your heart.

For more than a decade, doctors have warned that the affluent American diet, heavy on beef and other fat-rich foods, raises cholesterol levels and appears to be a major factor in causing coronary attacks.

But it's only in the last few years that researchers have found growing evidence linking the high-fat, low-fiber American diet with cancer of the breast and colon, which together strike about 180,000 Americans each year.

The intriguing clues have come from such widely separated spots on the globe as Africa and Japan. Diet, for example, may explain why an American woman is five times more likely to develop breast cancer than a woman living in Japan.

While the diet link with cancer leaves many questions yet to be answered, and debate swirls over whether too much fat or too little fiber is the most important for colon cancer, some leading experts believe that enough already is known to spur changes in the way most Americans eat.

"There already is plenty of reason to lower the fat content of our diet," explained Dr. Ernst L. Wynder of the American Health Foundation in New York, referring to the heart-attack risk. "The evidence (for the diet-cancer link) is growing," he added, and "being prudent means you don't have to have all the answers before acting."

Dr. Marvin Schneiderman of the National Cancer Institute put it this way: "What should I do? You do things on the basis of good, strong suspicion. And the good, strong suspicion now includes these dietary things."

Schneiderman has estimated that about 10,000 of the 42,000 annual American deaths from colon cancer, and at least some breast cancer deaths, could be prevented if all Americans switched to a safer diet.

He said this means reducing the consumption of beef and other fatty foods, and replacing this in the diet with more vegetables and fruits that have relatively high fiber (the nondigestible part of food) content.

This is what many nutritionists have been saying for years, even before the diet-cancer links began to be discovered several years ago. Experts now hope that future research will pin down more about just what diet may best protect against these and possibly some other types of cancer.

The heart-diet evidence, detailed in an earlier chapter, adds up to this: Saturated fats in meat can raise the level of cholesterol in the blood, and it's cholesterol that can gum up the coronary arteries to set the stage for a heart attack.

How could diet affect your risks of getting cancer? What evidence has made these and other cancer experts suggest that Americans eat less fat — and probably more fiber in the process?

Some of the evidence:

■ Most Japanese eat much less red meat than Americans, with rice and fish the big staples in their diets. The rate of colon cancer in Japan is only a fourth as high as in the United States; the rate for breast cancer only a fifth as high. But when Japanese men and women migrate to the United States and Americanize their eating habits, their rates for these types of cancer rise.

■ In the United States, Seventh Day Adventists, many of whom are vegetarians, were found in a large California study to have 10 percent less cancer of the colon and somewhat less cancer of the breast than other Californians.

■ The highest breast cancer rates are found in the Scandinavian countries, where the consumption of animal fats is very high.

■ In Israel, these same types of cancer are generally more common among Jews who have migrated from rich-diet America and Europe than those who have come from Asia and Africa.

■ In Africa, where fibrous foods make up the bulk of the diet, colon cancer is rare.

■ In animal experiments, cancer of both the breast and colon have been induced with high-fat diets.

The mechanisms through which diet may cause an increased risk of developing cancer still are debated. They probably work in an indirect way, but that makes them no less important.

Studies have found that American women tend to have high levels of various fatty substances, including cholesterol and cholesterol metabolites, in their breast fluids. This shows that what a woman eats can affect the chemicals that end up in her breasts. And it's known that cholesterol can be metabolized (converted) by the body into hormone-like chemicals, similar to some hormones linked to breast cancer in animals.

Other studies have shown that a high-fat diet can influence the amount of bile acid and cholesterol in the colon, and also may upset the equilibrium of the bacteria that are normally found there. The chemical changes may directly cause cancer, some experts theorize, or the bacteria can metabolize certain foods into cancer-causing chemicals.

Fiber in the diet may both dilute and speed up elimination of the contents of the intestinal tract, thereby preventing any chemical-causing substances (either eaten or made in the intestine) from having a chance to cause cancer.

All this, of course, is only circumstantial evidence. The diet-heart link is still debated, too, although stronger evidence has been gathered for it over many more years of study.

But don't worry about a conflict between the fiber theory and the fat theory.

"You can't separate them out," said Dr. Guy R. Newell, deputy director of the National Cancer Institute and head of its diet research program. For example, he said, "If you make your diet higher in fiber, you will unintentionally lower the fat. If you do one you will automatically do the other."

As you cut back on the amount of meat you eat, you probably will eat more fruits, vegetables, beans and possibly other foods high in fiber content such as whole-grain products. Bran is a particularly good source of fiber.

And don't worry that some of the cancer studies have come up with slightly different findings. Many of the these studies have specifically indicted animal fats, which tend to raise the level of the heart-villain cholesterol in the bloodstream. But other studies hint it may be the total fat content of the diet that people should worry about to reduce their cancer risk.

In either case, the prudent eating steps listed at the end of Chapter 2 are the right advice to follow. These steps are designed not only to lower your consumption of animal fats and cholesterol, but also to reduce the total amount of fat you eat as a way of keeping your weight under control.

So while all the advice at the end of Chapter 2 is good for cancer as well as heart concerns, here are a few particularly important tips applying to cancer prevention:

■ Eat more fish and poultry and less high-fat beef, lamb and pork.

■ When you do eat meat, choose lean cuts. Trim visible fat and discard the fat that cooks out.

■ Instead of whole milk and cheese made from whole milk and cream, use skimmed or low-fat milk and cheese.

■ At the same time, eat more fruits, vegetables and whole-grain products (for their relatively high fiber content) while consuming less meat.

Changing what you eat won't reduce your cancer risk overnight. Many questions remain, including how long it would take for the hoped-for benefits to reduce your cancer risk. Still, if you delay acting it will take just that much longer before any benefits start.

15/Catching cancer in time

Maybe you think there's only a remote chance that cancer will strike you — so why bother with early detection efforts? Actually, at current rates, 55 million Americans now living — one out of every four — will develop cancer sometime during his or her lifetime.

Or maybe you figure that if an early-detection test does find cancer, you'll just have to start worrying about it that much sooner.

So you tell yourself, "Don't borrow such scary trouble."

Just ask someone who has cancer what he or she thinks about the importance of finding cancer as early as possible. And consider odds like these:

When cancer of the colon is detected and treated in its early stages, seven out of every 10 patients are alive five years later. But too often it has spread to nearby lymph nodes when the person first sees a doctor, and that means the chance for survival already has dropped to about 45 percent. If the cancer has spread beyond these nodes, the chance for survival is much lower.

There are a number of ways to detect cancer early.

For colon cancer, there's the the proctoscopic ("procto") examination. For breast cancer, the monthly breast self-examination and periodic checks by a physician. For cervical cancer, the Pap test. And there are the Seven Warning Signals to alert you to possible signs of cancer.

Why don't people take advantage of these means to find out if anything is wrong?

"I think people tend to think they're immortal," said Dr. Frank Rauscher, senior vice president of the American Cancer Society. "Cancer isn't going to happen to me. It happens to somebody two blocks down the road. We just don't take advantage of the technology available."

Dr. Victor Gilbertsen, director of the University of Minnesota Hospitals' nationally noted Cancer Detection Center, looked at it this way:

"I really think, more than anything, it's a lack of information. A lot of people don't realize the success rate if cancer is found early, compared with the poor survival rate if found late."

The idea behind early detection is to catch the cancer early enough so that surgery (or, for some types of cancer, radiation treatment) can get rid of all of it — before it starts spreading. Any cancer cells that spread through the body can form the seeds of deadly new cancerous growths.

More than 20,000 people have participated in Gilbertsen's Cancer Detection Center program over the last 30 years. Many have returned for annual checks over the years. The success rates of this center often are cited by national experts to prove the value of early detection.

Here's a look at some of the major types of cancer and what can be done to reduce the nation's cancer toll:

Breast cancer: A monthly check

Breast cancer is the No. 1 cancer killer of American women. About 100,000 new cases are diagnosed annually and breast cancer takes the lives of about 34,000 women each year.

The experience at Gilbertsen's Cancer Detection Center has shown that annual physical examinations of the breast by the physician (even without an X-ray of the breasts, which is not routinely done there) plus monthly breast self-examinations by the woman can prevent many deaths.

Of the 118 women in the program who developed breast cancer over the three decades the center has operated, 102 were alive five years after the cancer was discovered — and most have had had no recurrence of their cancer. This is an 86 percent survival rate, compared with the national average rate of about 60 percent.

(Five-year survival statistics are the standard for cancer cases. While some types of cancer, including breast, may return after this time,

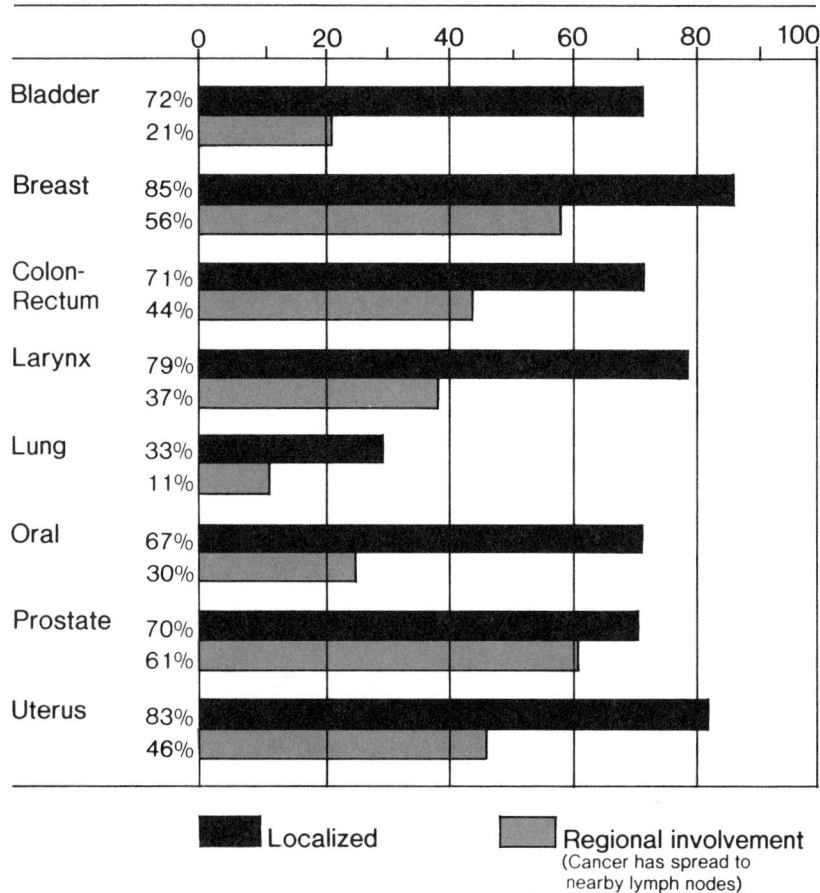

Five-year cancer survival rates for selected sites*

Site	Localized	Regional involvement
Bladder	72%	21%
Breast	85%	56%
Colon-Rectum	71%	44%
Larynx	79%	37%
Lung	33%	11%
Oral	67%	30%
Prostate	70%	61%
Uterus	83%	46%

■ Localized   ▨ Regional involvement (Cancer has spread to nearby lymph nodes)

*Adjusted for normal life expectancy, Source/End Results Group, National Cancer Institute

Chart shows increased survival rates when cancer is detected at the localized stage. Localized means there is no detectable sign of any spread beyond the organ where the cancer started. Regional means that cancer is found in nearby lymph nodes. The nodes serve as filters and may retard the spread for a while. But when the cancer has spread even this far, it increases the odds that some cancerous cells have spread through the body where they can form the seeds for new malignant tumors. If new tumors already have started appearing elsewhere in the body, the malignancy is advanced and chances of survival are extremely low for most types of cancer.

most people who reach the five-year mark are considered cured.)

Although more than 95 percent of all breast cancer appears in women after age 35, the American Cancer Society urges women to start breast self-examination in high school. This will allow very early detection of breast cancer and will make the woman familiar with her breasts so she can detect any suspicious change — a lump or thickening — that might occur later. X-ray checks of the breasts, except in special cases, aren't recommended until age 50.

Colon cancer: The preventive "procto"

Cancer of the colon and adjoining rectum account for 52,000 American deaths each year. It's the No. 2 cancer killer of both men (behind lung cancer) and women (behind breast cancer).

A "procto" exam involves inserting a proctoscope, which is a lighted tube, through the rectum into the lower part of the large intestine, where the majority of colon tumors develop. The cancer can actually be seen through this scope.

The "procto" also offers a way to "prevent" some colon cancer, Gilbertsen said. Here's what's involved:

Any polyps (small growths) found in the colon can be removed with an attachment on the scope, without surgery. Some of these polyps are precancerous, he said, and removing them stops the cancer process before it gets a chance to become full-fledged cancer.

By removing such polyps when they have been found, he said, only about half the normally expected colon cancer cases have occurred among patients getting annual exams at the center. Other researchers report similar results.

The American Cancer Society recommends "procto" exams for everyone 40 or older. Most colon cancer occurs after that age.

Despite the clear benefits of a "procto" exam, many people have shunned this sometimes uncomfortable procedure. So a new approach to detecting colon cancer early is being tried.

This occult-blood test can be done either as part of a regular checkup by the doctor, or the patient can use a special kit at home. In either case, a stool specimen is smeared on a slide. Then the slide is sent in for laboratory examination to see if there's any "occult," or invisible, blood that might indicate the presence of a cancerous growth in the intestinal tract.

The American Cancer Society endorses this test for use in addition to — but not as a substitute for — a "procto" check. The "procto" has proven benefits, but the blood tests can detect bleeding from a tumor higher in the colon than the "procto" can reach. Some studies indicate that 40 percent of colon cancers start at this higher level.

If blood is detected, extensive tests — including X-rays — are necessary to see if the bleeding is coming from a tumor or something else. The X-ray exam poses some risk from the radiation exposure, and all the tests together cost several hundred dollars.

Thus many experts want to know more about the potential value of the occult-blood test — and its limitations — before deciding how widely the test should be used. The key question: How often will hidden blood in the stool turn out to be from an ulcer or something else other than cancer?

Gilbertsen has recruited 48,000 Minnesotans between the ages of 50 and 80 for the largest test in the nation of this occult-blood test. In this 10-year study, which was fully under way in 1978, a third of the participants are receiving the blood test annually and a third every two years. The rest are relying on whatever steps their own doctors recommend.

In the first year, Gilbertsen reported, samples from 917 participants turned up evidence of hidden blood in the stool. Seventy-two of these people were found to have either colon cancer or, in a few cases, rectal cancer.

"Most of the cancers we found were at an early stage," Gilbertsen said. "The outlook would seem to be good for these people."

But he cautioned that it's too early to say anything definite about the value of the test. The pickup rate is not expected to be as high in succeeding years, since the first test might reveal tumors that had gone undetected for some time.

Uterine cancer: The Pap test

The simple Pap test can detect very early cancerous changes in the cervix (neck) of the uterus, before it's full-fledged cancer and when treatment is almost 100 percent successful.

The Pap test is given much of the credit for the 70-percent reduction in deaths from cancer of the uterus over the last 40 years. A pelvic examination at the same time can detect cancer of the body of the uterus or cancer of the ovary.

Still, about 7,400 American women die each year from cervical cancer, and 3,300 more from cancer of the endometrium (the lining of the body of the uterus).

"Uterine cancer could be reduced dramatically as a cause of death if every adult woman had a Pap test with her regular health checkup, and if every woman over 35 reported any abnormal bleeding promptly to her physician," says the American Cancer Society.

Prostate cancer: Find it early

Cancer of the prostate (a male gland located below the bladder) takes the lives of 21,000 Americans each year, making it the third leading cause of cancer deaths in American men.

This type of cancer can be detected by a doctor's gloved finger, feeling the prostate through the rectum. Most cancer of the prostate occurs in men over 60.

Lung cancer: Stop smoking

For the biggest cancer killer of all, lung cancer, cessation of cigarette smoking clearly remains the chief way to reduce that death toll. The survival rate for lung cancer is very low. Over-all, only one out of 10 persons with lung cancer is alive five years after it is diagnosed.

The regular checkup

How often should a person see a doctor for any early-detection tests?

Until a few years ago, the American Cancer Society urged "an annual checkup." Then, without fanfare, the society changed to recommend a "regular checkup."

American Cancer Society officials said they felt that the annual checkup was an easy-to-follow message that wouldn't create confusion. But now many experts say the frequency of the various cancer-detection tests should be based on a number of factors — age, occupation (as it relates to a number of types of cancer), family history of cancer and others.

Gilbertsen said that if full use were made of existing early detection methods, and there were no smoking to cause lung cancer, the nation's death toll from cancer probably could be about "cut in half."

This means that almost 200,000 American lives a year could be saved with what's already known about preventing lung cancer and catching many of the other major types of malignancies early.

What you should know:

The American Cancer Society lists Seven Warning Signals of possible cancer:

■ Unusual bleeding or discharge (particularly important for cancer of the uterus or colon).

■ A lump or thickening in the breast or elsewhere.

■ A sore that doesn't heal (particularly important for cancer in the mouth and for skin cancer.)

■ Change in bowel or bladder habits (for colon and prostate cancer).

■ Nagging hoarseness or cough (for cancer of the lung or throat).

■ Indigestion or difficulty in swallowing (for cancer of the stomach or esophagus).

■ Obvious change in a wart or mole (for skin cancer).

Quick call — or "watch and wait"?

Some of the symptoms — for example, suspected blood in the urine, or a worrisome lump for a woman who usually has a lump-free breast — call for a prompt check with a physician. But you can still phone first to describe the symptom and see if you need to come in for an office visit.

For some of the other symptoms, common sense must prevail. Every case of indigestion or coughing can't be read as a cancer warning. But the National Cancer Institute recommends that if any symptom on the list lasts more than two weeks, you should check with a doctor.

In most cases, these symptoms will turn out to be something other than cancer. But the only safe thing to do is to check.

Three "don'ts":

■ Don't wait for symptoms to become painful. Pain is not an early cancer sign, but typically comes later after the cancer has progressed too far to be removed successfully by surgery or destroyed by radiation.

■ Don't forget your mouth. It's a easy place to spot cancer — and also important, with 24,000 cases of oral cancer reported in the nation each year. If any suspicious signs occur in the mouth and last more than two weeks, they should be reported to a dentist or physician. These include changes in color, sores or bumps.

■ Don't let looking for symptoms replace the Pap test, "procto" and other available early-detection methods described in this chapter. They can often reveal cancer *before* symptoms develop — the best possible approach. The Seven Warning Signs are a second line of defense — but knowing them could still save your life.

Breast self-examination

Step 1

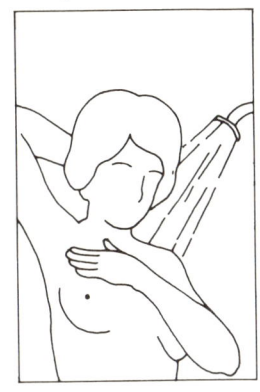

Step 2

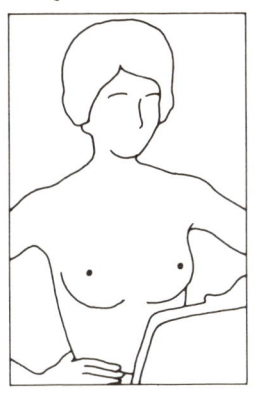

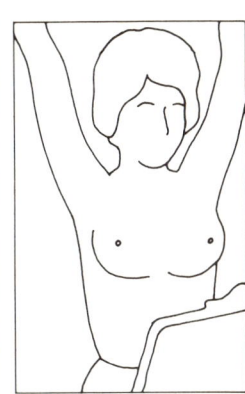

Step 3

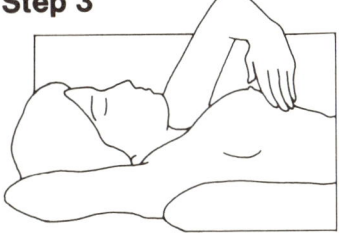

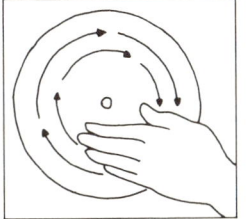

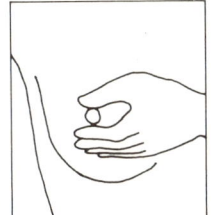

Here's what the American Cancer Society recommends for monthly breast self-examination:

Step 1: Examine your breasts during bath or shower; hands glide easier over wet skin. With fingers flat, move gently over every part of each breast. Check for any lump, hard knot or thickening.

Step 2: Inspect your breasts with arms at your sides. Then raise your arms overhead. Look for any changes in contour of each breast, a swelling, dimpling of skin or changes in the nipple. Then rest palms on hips and press down firmly to flex your chest muscles. (In most women, left and right breasts don't exactly match.)

Step 3: To examine your right breast, put a pillow or folded towel under your right shoulder. Place right hand behind your head to distribute breast tissue more evenly on the chest. Using your left hand, fingers flat, press gently in small circular motions around an imaginary clock face. A ridge of firm tissue in the lower curve of each breast is normal. Then move in an inch, toward nipple, and keep circling to examine every part of your breast; this will require at least three more circles. Repeat procedure on your left breast. Finally, gently squeeze the nipple of each breast and look for any discharge, clear or bloody.

Check with your doctor if you find any suspicious lump, other abnormality or discharge. For women who menstruate the best time to do the self-examination is a week after the start of the period.

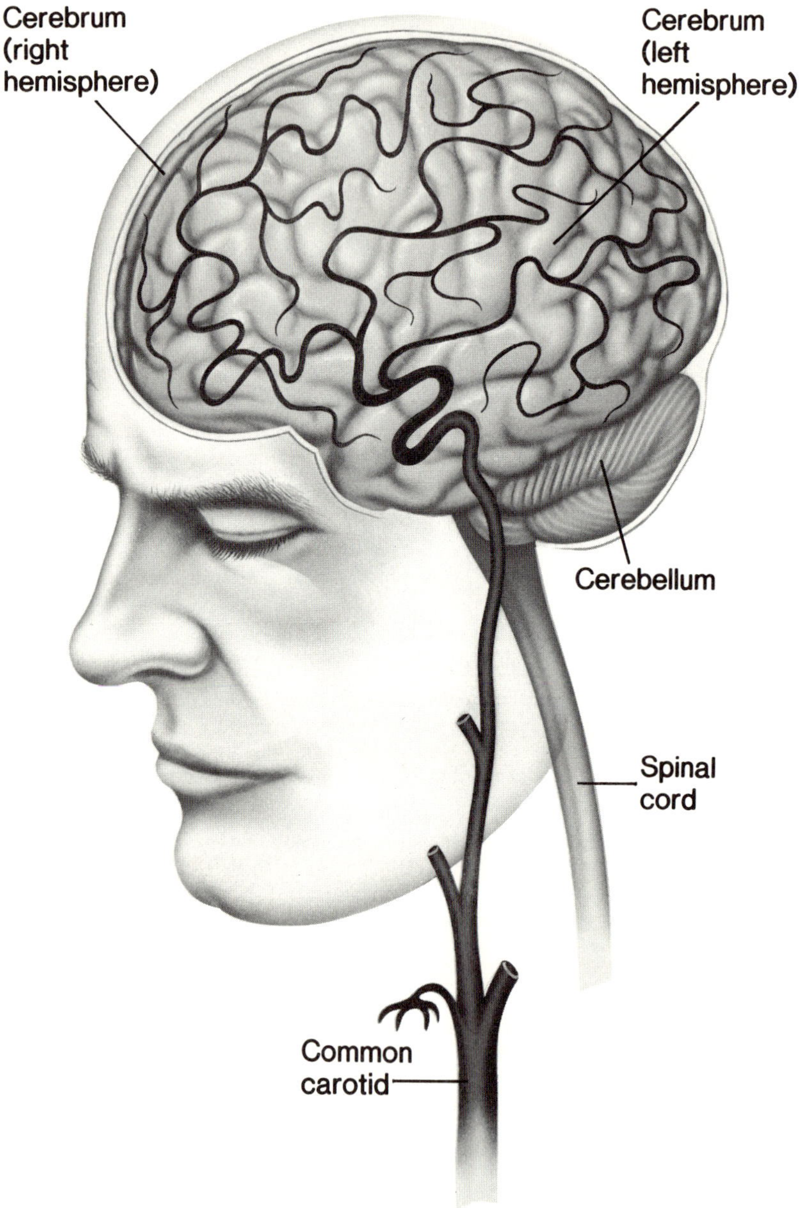
Cerebrum
(right
hemisphere)
Cerebrum
(left
hemisphere)
Cerebellum
Spinal
cord
Common
carotid

Strokes/ Attacks on the brain

A stroke is a close cousin to a heart attack — but it strikes the brain rather than the heart.

In the typical stroke, a blood clot interrupts the normal flow of blood into a section of the brain and tissue there dies. Thus the process is similar to a clot in a coronary artery that triggers a heart attack. In a small percentage of strokes, however, a blood vessel in the brain ruptures, causing a hemorrhagic stroke.

Smoking, diet-related high levels of cholesterol in the blood and high blood pressure have been linked to increased risks of both strokes and heart attacks. In strokes, however, high blood pressure is most important.

Not only do strokes take the lives of some 170,000 Americans each year, but they leave many others with varying degrees of disability. Strokes can cause partial paralysis in the arm and leg on one side of the body, or difficulty in speaking, or loss of memory, or a combination of problems. Early rehabilitation often helps to reduce these after-effects, but strokes remain a major crippler as well as killer.

So the big hope is prevention. In addition to watching blood pressure and taking other actions that may reduce the chance of a stroke as well as a heart attack, there's a second line of defense. That's what the next chapter is about.

16/Vision blurry? Arm numb?

Grace Anderson was watching TV when "all of a sudden I noticed my vision was getting fuzzy."

She instinctively put her right hand up to her face, covering her right eye in the process.

"I couldn't see a thing — I was completely blind in the left eye," she recalled.

She took a quick nap, and when she awoke about 45 minutes later, everything was fine.

Or was it?

Morris Frederick was driving down the road one day when suddenly he noticed his left hand was numb.

But the numbness lasted only a few minutes. He thought no more about it.

The next day, when he started to make a cup of tea, he picked the kettle off the stove only to have it slip through his hand and drop back onto the stove with a clatter. His entire left arm, from fingers to shoulder, was numb.

The numbness lasted only about an hour.

Then he was all right.

Or was he?

"Most people would never see a doctor with these symptoms — because the symptoms go away," said Dr. A. B. Baker, head of the neurology program at Mount Sinai Hospital in Minneapolis and an international authority on strokes.

Fortunately, Frederick and Anderson saw their doctors. Their lives were at stake. Alerting the public to recognize these and similar telltale symptoms is now seen as a way to lower dramatically the high toll of death and disability from strokes.

Anderson, 81 at the time, and Frederick, 69, had suffered "little strokes." Technically these aren't real strokes at all, because the symptoms pass quickly without leaving any actual brain damage. But they show that the stage has been set for a disabling or killer stroke — unless the person gets proper drugs or surgery to correct the trouble.

The stakes are high.

Full-fledged strokes hit an estimated half-million Americans each year. About 170,000 of them die, making this the nation's No. 3 killer, behind only heart attacks and cancer. Most of the survivors are left with varying degrees of paralysis or other problems affecting brain functions, including speech and eyesight.

"We can make a big dent in these awesome figures," said Baker in urging public awareness of the quickly vanishing symptoms that can be harbingers of a killing or crippling stroke.

The villain in strokes is blood clots.

As a person becomes older, the arteries leading up through the neck to the brain often become more and more clogged with fatty deposits which narrow these blood vessels. Blood clots then begin to form at these roughened spots.

You have two pencil-sized carotid arteries going up the front of your neck and two somewhat smaller arteries going up the back of your head. Think of them as rivers of blood. Within your skull, these "rivers" branch out into many smaller blood vessels, or "streams," that carry nourishing blood to the billions of cells in your brain.

If a big chunk of the clot breaks away and floats "downstream" into the brain, where it dams up one of the smaller vessels, blood can't get through. Within minutes, brain cells begin to die in the blood-starved area of the brain. This is a full-fledged stroke that can kill or cripple.

Fortunately, chances are very good that little strokes will occur first and provide a warning.

What typically happens, Baker explained, is that only a tiny particle breaks off from a growing clot. It floats into the brain and clogs a blood vessel there. But this tiny clot-particle may dissolve before brain damage results. Or enough other blood may get into that small section of brain from other arteries to prevent any lasting damage.

Still, the temporary interruption of normal blood flow caused by this breakaway tiny clot-particle is enough to cause the symptoms of a little stroke — and warn that a full-fledged stroke may strike soon, although there's no way of knowing when it may occur.

After little strokes start, Baker noted, they usually recur. Frederick had his two warning episodes in a two-day period, which puzzled him enough to go to a hospital to seek the cause. Anderson continued to have a number of little strokes that caused her left eye to go blind temporarily and one that had the same effect on her right eye, even after she was hospitalized for observation.

Here's why detecting those little strokes is so important:

■ Studies have indicated that at least 40 percent of all people who suffer full-fledged strokes have had one or more little strokes, often within the past month. The percentage may be much higher.

"I'm convinced there are a large number of patients who have little strokes and don't even remember them," Baker said, because the symptoms are so fleeting and the public hasn't been alerted to recognize them.

■ Other studies show that about 50 percent of people who have little strokes, at least when they have more than one, go on to have full-fledged strokes — unless they see a doctor. With proper surgical or drug treatment, as their particular case may require, "most can be helped," said Baker.

Anderson and Frederick both had such extensive obstructions that they were almost certain candidates for major strokes, Baker said.

Both Anderson and Frederick underwent surgery to remove large clots and open up the carotid arteries in their necks.

"That will last another 81 years," Baker joked with Anderson after her surgery. She had two operations, one on her right carotid artery, the other on her left, just below where these arteries run up under the jawbone. Each operation took about two hours from start to finish, although the actual cleaning out of the carotid artery takes only about 20 minutes.

Frederick needed an operation on only the right side of his neck. The nerve pathways from most parts of the body cross over before entering the brain. Therefore, the little strokes that affected his *left* arm showed that a section in the *right* half of his brain had been denied sufficient blood flow for a brief period. And the cause was clotting in the *right* carotid artery in his neck.

Special X-rays are used to locate a clot, with dye injected into the arteries to make the clot stand out. Depending on the general condition of the patient and other factors, one of three approaches is used:

■ When the obstruction is in an accessible area in the neck, which frequently is the case, the relatively simple surgical operation that Anderson and Frederick had is used.

■ If the clotting is above the point where the scalpel can reach to remove the obstruction, drugs that greatly reduce the normal clotting properties of blood are used. There are several such drugs, one of which is being used more and more — simple aspirin.

■ In carefully selected cases, some neurosurgeons are now actually operating on the brain. This still relatively rare operation connects a scalp artery into a brain artery to provide a new source of blood flow. This operation is similar in purpose to the so-called coronary bypass surgery now used to treat many heart patients.

So anything from aspirin to brain surgery may help, depending on the specific case. Why aspirin?

The blood has red blood cells (which carry oxygen), white blood cells (which fight infection) and tiny plate-shaped platelets (which break open when they hit a wound or rough spot in a blood vessel, releasing a substance that causes blood to clot).

Among the many things it does in the body, aspirin reduces the platelets' ability to stick to a blood vessel and start the clotting mechanism.

But Baker cautioned that anyone suffering little strokes should not decide on his or her own to use aspirin. Aspirin may not be what's needed in an individual case, and too much aspirin sometimes causes bleeding problems in the stomach.

A technical term often used for a little stroke is transient ischemic attack, usually just called TIA, explained Baker. Transient means it quickly passes; ischemic means a section of tissue is denied ample blood.

Some doctors say that they shouldn't be called little strokes at all, since they leave no lasting brain damage. But whether called TIAs or little strokes, recognizing them as an early-warning signal of impending trouble offers a new hope for saving the lives or health for many thousands of Americans.

What you should know:

One or more of the following symptoms can provide an early-warning signal that the person should seek medical help to head off a possible stroke:

■ Temporary weakness or numbness of the face, arm and leg on one side of the body. This sometimes causes a stumbling gait.

■ Temporary loss of speech, or difficulty in speaking or difficulty in understanding speech.

■ Temporary dimness or loss of vision, particularly in one eye.

■ Unexplained dizziness, usually associated with double vision.

Dr. Baker of Mount Sinai Hospital said that these "warning episodes:"

■ Typically last anywhere from a minute to an hour, but may last from a few seconds to 24 hours.

■ Have a sudden onset.

■ Tend to recur with the same general pattern. That is, if you have a weakness on one side of your body, it's likely to recur on that side — although the first time it may be in the arm, the next time in the leg.

■ Occur most frequently in older people, typically over age 65, but can occur in a person of any age.

What to do

What should you do if you or someone you know has any one of these symptoms? Baker suggests:

■ If you're puzzled by what happens — for example, you think an arm or a leg is more than just "going to sleep" on you — it's best to check with a doctor even the first time that you have such symptoms.

■ If there's recurrence, don't delay, said Baker. Your life may depend on it.

■ Don't forego seeking help because you are young. Even if you're young, these symptoms either indicate you're vulnerable to a stroke or you may have some other neurological problem that needs attention.

The hemorrhagic stroke is different

The early warning signs above all indicate that the stage is being set for the type of stroke caused by a clot. A much less common type of stroke is caused by a blood vessel in the brain rupturing.

■ Possible signs of a developing hemorrhagic stroke are a very severe headache accompanied by a stiff neck. This should alert a person to contact a physician immediately.

Appendix A/
Canadian lifestyle quiz

The Canadian government, a leader in the health prevention field, developed this easy-to-take quiz that shows how your lifestyle affects your health.

While some heart experts might wish the nutrition questions took cholesterol into consideration, this quiz covers a surprising amount of territory. It includes not only heart, cancer and stroke risk factors, but also asks questions relating to four more of the top 12 causes of deaths in this country. Accidents are No. 4. Diabetes, No. 6, is more common among people who are overweight. Alcohol abuse can lead to cirrhosis of the liver, the nation's seven-ranked cause of death. And smoking can lead to emphysema, No. 12.

Your lifestyle profile

— Indicate by checking only the boxes that apply to you.
— The plus (+) and minus (—) signs next to some numbers indicate more than (+) and less than (—).

Exercise

	Heavy physical, walking, housework	Desk work	
Amount of physical effort expended during the workday: mostly	[1]	[3]	

	Daily	Weekly	Seldom
Participation in physical activities—(skiing, golf, swimming, etc.) (lawn mowing, gardening, etc.)?	[1]	[3]	[5]

	3 times weekly	Weekly	Seldom
Participation in a vigorous exercise program?	[1]	[3]	[5]

	1+	—1	None
Average miles walked or jogged per day?	[1]	[3]	[5]

	10+	—10	
Flights of stairs climbed per day?	[1]	[3]	

Nutrition

	No	5 to 19 lbs.	20+ lbs.
Are you overweight?	[1]	[3]	[5]

	Each Day	3 times weekly	
Do you eat a wide variety of foods—something from each of the following five food groups: (1) meat, fish, poultry, dried legumes, eggs or nuts; (2) milk or milk products; (3) bread or cereals; (4) fruits; (5) vegetables?	[1]	[3]	

Alcohol

	0 to 7	8 to 15	16+
Average bottles (12 oz.) of beer per week?	1	3	5
Average number of hard liquor (1½ oz.) drinks per week?	1	3	5
Average number of glasses (5 oz.) of wine or cider per week?	1	3	5
Total number of drinks per week, including beer, liquor and wine?	1	3	5

Drugs

	No		Yes
Do you take drugs illegally?	1		5
Do you consume alcoholic beverages together with certain drugs (tranquilizers, barbiturates, antihistamines or illegal drugs)?	1		5
Do you use pain-killers improperly or excessively?	1		5

Tobacco

	None	—10	10+
Cigarettes smoked per day?	1	3	5

	None	—5	5+
Cigars smoked per day?	1	3	5

	None	—2	2+
Pipe tobacco pouches per week?	1	3	5

Personal health

	Seldom	Occasionally	Frequently
Do you experience periods of depression?	1	3	5

	No	Occasionally	Frequently
Does anxiety interfere with your daily activities?	1	3	5

	Yes	No	
Do you get enough satisfying sleep?	1	3	
Are you aware of the causes and dangers of VD?	1	3	

	Monthly	Occasionally	
Breast self-examination? (If not applicable, do not score.)	1	3	

Road and water safety

	—10,000	10,000+	
Mileage per year as driver or passenger?	1	3	

	No	by 10 mph+	by 20 mph+
Do you often exceed the speed limit?	1	3	5

	Always	Occasionally	Never
Do you wear a seatbelt?	[1]	[3]	[5]

	No	Yes	
Do you drive a motorcycle, moped or snowmobile?	[1]	[3]	

	Yes		No
If yes to the above, do you always wear a regulation safety helmet?	[1]		[5]

	Never		Occasionally
Do you ever drive under the influence of alcohol?	[1]		[5]

	Never		Occasionally
Do you ever drive when your ability may be affected by drugs?	[1]		[5]

	Yes	No	
Are you aware of water safety rules?	[1]	[3]	

	Yes	No	
If you participate in water sports or boating, do you wear a life jacket? (If not applicable, do not score.)?	[1]	[3]	

General

	0 to 1	1 to 4	4+
Average time watching TV per day (in hours)?	[1]	[3]	[5]

	Yes	No	
Are you familiar with first-aid procedures?	[1]	[3]	

	No	Occasionally	Yes
Do you ever smoke in bed?	[1]	[3]	[5]

	Yes	Occasionally	No
Do you always make use of clothing and equipment provided for your safety at work? (If not applicable, do not score.)	[1]	[3]	[5]

Add up the number of checks you have in each column:

Column 1: _____ checks x 1 point each = _____ points

Column 2: _____ checks x 3 points each = _____ points

Column 3: _____ checks x 5 points each = _____ points

Your total score _____ **points**

Here's what Health and Welfare Canada says about your score:

34 to 45, Excellent

"Congratulations! Excellent indicates you have a commendable lifestyle based on sensible habits and a lively awareness of personal health. Keep up the good work and maintain this rating."

46 to 55, Good

"You have a sound grasp of basic health principles. Only one to 10 points separate you from the elite. With a minimum of change you can develop an excellent lifestyle pattern. Make the effort to move up to 'Excellent' and stay there.

56 to 65, Risky

"You are taking unnecessary risks with your health. Several of your lifestyle habits are based on unwise personal choices which should be changed if potential health problems are to be avoided. Look at your test again. A few common-sense decisions can mean a 'Good' rating, but the challenge is to move your lifestyle up to 'Excellent'."

66 or more, Hazardous

"A 'hazardous' rating indicates a high-risk lifestyle. This is a danger zone — but even hazardous lifestyles can be modified and potential health problems overcome. All it takes is a little conscientious effort to improve basic living patterns. Start making those improvements right now."

(The question about television may surprise you. However, Hank Leclair of the Information Directorate at Health and Welfare Canada, which developed the test, said "the longer you watch TV, the less time you have to play tennis or ski or have other physicial activities to keep in shape.")

Appendix B/
12 leading causes of death

The 12 leading causes of death in 1978 in the United States, as reported by the U.S. Public Health Service's National Center for Health Statistics:

1. Heart disease

    Heart attacks 637,270

    Other heart disease 84,830

    Total 722,100

2. Cancer 394,480

3. Strokes 171,480

4. Accidents 103,740

5. Influenza and pneumonia 57,980

6. Diabetes 32,580

7. Cirrhosis of liver 29,720

8. Arteriosclerosis (hardening of arteries) 29,020

9. Suicide 25,770

10. Certain causes of death in early infancy

    (including birth injuries and immaturity) 22,310

11. Homicides 19,910

12. Emphysema 15,870

Other causes of death 288,790

Total deaths **1,913,750**

Appendix C/
For more information...

American Heart Association affiliates across the nation offer pamphlets and other material on a wide variety of heart topics. This information includes guides for lowering cholesterol levels and brochures on high blood pressure and other aspects of heart-attack prevention. The heart association also is a good place to check for information on cardio-pulmonary resuscitation (CPR) classes.

American Cancer Society chapters offer booklets and other information on various aspects of cancer, including early-detection and smoking cessation. Some chapters hold quit-smoking classes.

You can contact a Mental Health Association chapter for a copy of the booklet "How to Deal With Your Tensions."

The National Cancer Institute sponsors a network of Cancer Information Service toll-free phone services that provide information on cancer.

Here's a listing of these four sources of further information:

American Heart Association

National center: 7320 Greenville Av., Dallas, Texas, 75231

Affiliates by regions

Great Plains region:

Dakota Affiliate, 1005 12th Av. SE., Jamestown, N.D., 58401

Iowa Heart Association, 3810 Ingersoll Av., Des Moines, Iowa, 50312

Kansas Affiliate, 5229 W. 7th St., Topeka, Kan., 66606

Minnesota Affiliate, 4701 W. 77th St., Minneapolis, Minn., 55435

Missouri Affiliate, 601 E. Broadway, Columbia, Mo., 65201

Nebraska Heart Association, 3624 Farnam, Omaha, Neb., 68134

Middle Atlantic region:

Maryland Affiliate, 10 South St., Suite 100, Baltimore, Md., 21202

North Carolina Heart Association, 1 Heart Circle, Chapel Hill, N.C., 27514

South Carolina Heart Association, 5868 Percival Road, Columbia, S.C., 29260

Virginia Affiliate, 316 E. Clay St., Richmond, Va., 23219

Nation's Capital Affiliate, 2233 Wisconsin Av. NW, Washington, D.C., 20007

West Virginia Affiliate, 211 35th St. SE, Charleston, W. Va., 25304

New England region:

Connecticut Affiliate, 71 Parker Av., Meriden, Conn., 06450

Maine Affiliate, 20 Winter St., Augusta, Me., 04330

Massachusetts Affiliate, 33 Broad St., Boston, Mass., 02109

New Hampshire Heart Association, 54 S. State St., Concord, N.H., 03301

Rhode Island Affiliate, 40 Broad St., Pawtucket, R.I., 02860

Vermont Heart Association, 56 Church St., Rutland, Vt., 05701

North Central region:

Chicago Heart Association, 20 N. Wacker, Chicago, Ill., 60606

Illinois Heart Association, 1181 N. Dirksen Parkway, Springfield, Ill., 62708

Indiana Affiliate, 222 S. Downey, Suite 222, Indianapolis, Ind., 46219

Kentucky Heart Association, 207 Speed Building, 333 Guthrie St., Louisville, Ky., 40202

Michigan Heart Association, 16310 W. Twelve Mile Road, Southfield, Mich., 48076

Northeast Ohio Affiliate, 1689 E. 115th St., Cleveland, Ohio, 44106

Ohio Affiliate, 10 E. Town St., Room 506, Columbus, Ohio, 43215

Wisconsin Affiliate, 795 N. Van Buren St., Milwaukee, Wis., 53202

Northwest-Rocky Mountain region:

Alaska Heart Association, 2330 E. 42nd St., Anchorage, Alaska, 99504

Colorado Heart Association, 4521 E. Virginia Av., Denver, Colo., 80222

Idaho Heart Association, 1301 S. Capitol Blvd., Boise, Idaho, 83706

Montana Heart Association, Prof. Bldg., 510 1st Av. N., Great Falls, Mont., 59401

Oregon Heart Association, 1500 SW 12th Av., Portland, Ore., 97201

Utah Heart Association, 250 E. 1st S., Salt Lake City, Utah, 84111

American Heart Association of **Washington** State, 333 First Av. W., Seattle, Wash., 98119

Wyoming Heart Association, 217 W. 18th St., Cheyennne, Wyo., 82001

Southern region:

Alabama Affiliate, 1449 Medical Park Drive., Birmingham, Ala., 35213

Arkansas Affiliate, 909 W. 2nd St., Little Rock, Ark., 72201

Florida Affiliate, 2828 Central Av., St. Petersburg, Fla., 33712

Georgia Heart Association, Broadview Plaza, Level C, 2581 Piedmont Rd., NE, Atlanta, Ga., 30324

Louisiana Affiliate, 3303 Tulane Av., New Orleans, La., 70119

Mississippi Affiliate, 4830 E. McWillie Circle, Jackson, Miss., 39206

Oklahoma Affiliate, 800 NE 15th St., Oklahoma City, Okla., 73111

Tennessee Affiliate, Suite 308, 1720 West End Building, Nashville, Tenn., 37203

Southwest region:

Arizona Affiliate, 1445 E. Thomas, Phoenix, Ariz., 85014

California Affiliate, 805 Burlway Road, Burlingame, Calif., 94010

American Heart Association of **Hawaii**, 245 N. Kukui St., Honolulu, Hawaii, 96817

Greater **Los Angeles** Affiliate, 2405 W. 8th St., Los Angeles, Calif., 90057

Nevada Affiliate, 455 W. 5th St., Reno, Nev., 89503

New Mexico Affiliate, 142 Truman St. NE, Suite D, Albuquerque, N.M., 87108

Texas Affiliate, 860 N. Highway 183, Austin, Texas, 78761

Upper Atlantic region:

Delaware Heart Association, Independence Mall, Suite 46, 1601 Concord Pike, Wilmington, Del., 19803

New Jersey Affiliate, 1525 Morris Av., Union, N.J., 07083

New York Heart Association, 205 E. 42nd St., New York, N.Y., 10017

New York State Affiliate, 3 W. 29th St., New York, N.Y., 10001

Pennsylvania Affiliate, 2743 N. Front St., Harrisburg, Pa., 17100

Puerto Rico Heart Association, 554 Cabo Alverio St., Hato Rey Station, San Juan, Puerto Rico, 00919

American Cancer Society

National headquarters: **777 Third Av., New York, N.Y. 10017.**

Division offices

Alabama Division, 2926 Central Av., Birmingham, Ala. 35209

Alaska Division, 1343 G. St., Anchorage, Alaska, 99501

Arizona Division, 634 W. Indian School Road, P.O. Box 33187, Phoenix, Ariz., 85067

Arkansas Division, 5520 W. Markham St., P.O. Box 3822, Little Rock, Ark., 72203

California Division, 731 Market St., San Francisco, Calif., 94103

Colorado Division, 1809 E. 18th Av., P.O. Box 18268, Denver, Colo., 80218

Connecticut Division, Barnes Park South, 14 Village Lane, Wallingford., Conn., 06492

Delaware Division, Academy of Medicine Building, 1925 Lovering Av., Wilmington, Del., 19806

District of Columbia Division, Universal Building South, 1825 Connecticut Av., NW, Washington, D.C., 20009

Florida Division, 1001 S. MacDill Av., Tampa, Fla., 33609

Georgia Division, 2025 Peachtree Road NE, Suite 14, Atlanta, Ga., 30309

Hawaii Division, Community Services Center Building, 200 N. Vineyard Boulevard, Honolulu, Hawaii, 96817

Idaho Division, 1609 Abbs St., P.O. Box 5386, Boise, Idaho, 83705

Illinois Division, 37 S. Wabash Av., Chicago, Ill., 60603

Indiana Division, 2702 E. 55th Place, Indianapolis, Ind., 46220

Iowa Division, Highway 18 West, P.O. Box 980, Mason City, Iowa, 50401

Kansas Division, 3003 Van Buren St., Topeka, Kan., 66611

Kentucky Division, Medical Arts Building, 1169 Eastern Parkway, Louisville, Ky., 40217

Louisiana Division, Masonic Temple Building, Room 810, 333 St. Charles Av., New Orleans, La., 70130

Maine Division, Federal and Green Sts., Brunswick, Maine, 04011

Maryland Division, 200 E. Joppa Road, Towson, Md., 21204

Massachusetts Division, 247 Commonwealth Av., Boston, Mass. 02116

Michigan Division, 1205 E. Saginaw St., Lansing, Mich., 48906

Minnesota Division, 2750 Park Av., Minneapolis, Minn., 55407

Mississippi Division, 345 North Mart Plaza, Jackson, Miss., 39206

Missouri Division, 715 Jefferson St., P.O. Box 1066, Jefferson City, Mo., 65101

Montana Division, 2820 First Av. S., Billings, Mont., 59101

Nebraska Division, Overland Wolfe Centre, 6910 Pacific St., Suite 210, Omaha, Neb., 68106

Nevada Division, 953-35B E. Sahara, Suite 101 ST&P Building, Las Vegas, Nev., 89104

New Hampshire Division, 22 Bridge St., Manchester, N.H., 03101

New Jersey Division, 2700 Route 22, P.O. Box 1220, Union, N.J., 07083

New Mexico Division, 525 San Pedro NE, Albuquerque, N.M., 87108

New York State Division, 6725 Lyons St., P.O. Box 7, East Syracuse, N.Y., 13057

   Long Island Division, 535 Broad Hollow Road (Route 110), Melville, N.Y. 11746

   New York City Division, 19 W. 56th St., New York, N.Y., 10019

   Queens Division, 111-15 Queens Boulevard, Forest Hills, N.Y., 11375

   Westchester Division, 246 N. Central Av., Hartsdale, N.Y., 10530

North Carolina Division, 222 N. Person St., P.O. Box 27624, Raleigh, N.C., 27611

North Dakota Division, Hotel Graver Annex Building, 115 Roberts St., P.O. Box 426, Fargo, N.D., 58102

Ohio Division, 453 Lincoln Building, 1367 E. Sixth St., Cleveland, Ohio, 44114

Oklahoma Division, 1312 NW 24th St., Oklahoma City, Okla., 73106

Oregon Division, 910 NE Union Av., Portland, Ore., 97232

Pennsylvania Division, 3309 Spring St., P.O. Box 4175, Harrisburg, Pa., 17111

Philadelphia Division, 21 S. 12th St., Philadelphia, Pa., 19107

Puerto Rico Division, (Avenue Domenech 273 Hato Rey, P.R.), GPO Box 6004, San Juan, Puerto Rico, 00936

Rhode Island Division, 345 Blackstone Blvd., Providence, R.I., 02906

South Carolina Division, 2442 Devine St., Columbia, S.C., 29205

South Dakota Division, 700 S. 4th Av., Sioux Falls, S.D., 57104

Tennessee Division, 2519 White Av., Nashville, Tenn., 37204

Texas Division, 3834 Spicewood Springs Road, P.O. Box 9863, Austin, Texas, 78766

Utah Division, 610 East South Temple, Salt Lake City, Utah, 84102

Vermont Division, 13 Loomis St., Drawer C, Montpelier, Vt., 05602

Virginia Division, 3218 West Cary St., P.O. Box 7288, Richmond, Va., 23221

Washington Division, 323 First Av. W., Seattle, Wash., 98119

West Virginia Division, Suite 100, 240 Capital St., Charleston, W. Va., 25301

Wisconsin Division, 611 N. Sherman Av., P.O. Box 1626, Madison, Wis., 53701

Milwaukee Division, 6401 W. Capitol Drive, Milwaukee, Wis., 53216

Wyoming Division, Indian Hills Center, 506 Shoshoni, Cheyenne, Wyo., 82001

Cancer Information Service

Toll-free numbers for the Cancer Information Service, sponsored by the National Cancer Institute, are:

Alaska: 1-800-638-6070

California: From Area Codes (213), (714) and (805) 1-800-252-9066

Colorado: 1-800-332-1850

Connecticut: 1-800-922-0824

Delaware: 1-800-523-3586

District of Columbia: (Includes suburban Maryland and Northern Virginia) 232-2833

Florida: 1-800-432-5953

   Dade County: 547-6920

Hawaii: Oahu: 536-0111 (Neighbor Islands: Ask operator for Enterprise 6702)

Illinois: 800-972-0586

   Chicago: 346-9813

Kentucky: 800-432-9321

Maine: 1-800-225-7034

Maryland: 800-492-1444

Massachusetts: 1-800-952-7420

Minnesota: 1-800-582-5262

Montana: 1-800-525-0231

New Hampshire: 1-800-225-7034

New Jersey: 800-523-3586

New Mexico: 1-800-525-0231
New York: New York State: 1-800-462-7255
  Erie County: 845-4400
  New York City: 794-7982
North Carolina: 800-672-0943
  Durham County: 286-2266
Ohio: 1-800-282-6522
Pennsylvania: 1-800-822-3963
Texas: 1-800-392-2040
  Houston: 792-3245
Vermont: 1-800-225-7034
Washington: 1-800-552-7212
Wisconsin: 1-800-362-8038
Wyoming: 1-800-525-0231
Elsewhere in United States: 1-800-638-6694

(In most but not all areas of the nation, you must dial 1 before using a toll-free 800 number. If the number listed doesn't start with a 1 and your call doesn't go through, try it with the 1.)

Mental Health Association

National headquarters: 1800 N. Kent St., Arlington, Va., 22209

Division offices

Mental Health Association in **Alabama**, 306 Whitman St., Montgomery, Ala., 36104

Alaska Mental Health Association, 5531 Arctic Boulevard, Anchorage, Alaska, 99502

Mental Health Association in **Arizona**, 341 W. McDowell Road, Phoenix, Ariz., 85003

Mental Health Association in **Arkansas**, 121 E. Fourth St., Little Rock, Ark., 72201

Mental Health Association in **California**, 901 H St., Suite 212, Sacramento, Calif., 95814

Mental Health Association in **Colorado**, 252 Clayton St., Garden Level 2, Denver, Colo., 80206

Mental Health Association in **Connecticut**, 56 Arbor St., Hartford, Conn., 06106

Mental Health Association in **Delaware**, 1813 N. Franklin St., Wilmington, Del., 19802

District of Columbia Mental Health Association, 2101 16th St. NW., Washington, D.C. 20009

Mental Health Association of **Florida**, Suite 207, Myrick Building, 132 E. Colonial Drive, Orlando, Fla., 32801

Mental Health Association in **Georgia**, 100 Edgewood Av. NE, No. 502, Atlanta, Ga., 30303

Mental Health Association in **Hawaii**, 200 N. Vineyard Boulevard, Room 101, Honolulu, Hawaii, 96817

Idaho Mental Health Association, 3105½ State St., Boise, Idaho, 83703

Mental Health Association in **Illinois**, 103 N. Fifth St., Room 304, Springfield, Ill., 62701

Mental Health Association in **Indiana**, 1433 N. Meridian St., Indianapolis, Ind., 46202

Iowa Association for Mental Health, 315 E. Fifth St., Des Moines, Iowa, 50309

Mental Health Association in **Kansas**, 1205 Harrison St., Topeka, Kan., 66612

Kentucky Association for Mental Health, Suite 106, 310 West Liberty St., Louisville, Ky., 40202

Louisiana Association for Mental Health, 1528 Jackson Av., New Orleans, La., 70130

Maryland Association for Mental Health, 325 E. 25th St., Baltimore, Md., 21218

Massachusetts Association for Mental Health, 14 Somerset St., Boston, Mass., 02108

Mental Health Association in **Michigan**, 27208 Southfield Road, Lathrup Village, Mich., 48076

Mental Health Association in **Minnesota**, 6715 Minnetonka Blvd., Room 209-210, St. Louis Park, Minn., 55426

Mississippi Association for Mental Health, P.O. Box 5041, Jackson, Miss., 39216

Mental Health Association in **Missouri**, 129 E. Miller, Jefferson City, Mo., 65101

Mental Health Association in **Montana**, 201 S. Last Chance Gulch, Helena, Mont., 59601

New Jersey Association for Mental Health, 60 S. Fullerton Av., Montclair, N.J., 07042

New York State Association for Mental Health, 250 W. 57th St., Room 1425, New York, N.Y., 10019

Mental Health Association in **North Carolina**, 3701 National Drive, Suite 222, Raleigh, N.C., 27612

North Dakota Mental Health Association, Kirkwood Office Tower, 7th and Arbor Av., Bismark, N.D., 58501

Mental Health Association in **Ohio**, Suite 2440, 50 W. Broad St., Columbus, Ohio, 43215

Mental Health Association in **Oklahoma**, 3113 Classen Boulevard, Oklahoma City, Okla., 73118

Mental Health Association in **Oregon**, 718 W. Burnside, Room 301, Portland, Ore., 97209

Mental Health Association in **Pennsylvania**, 1207 Chestnut St., Philadelphia, Pa., 19107

Mental Health Association in **Rhode Island**, 55 Hope St., Providence, R.I., 02906

South Carolina Mental Health Association, 1823 Gadsden St., Columbia, S.C., 29201

South Dakota Mental Health Association, 101½ S. Pierre St., Box 355, Pierre, S.D., 57501

Tennessee Mental Health Association, 444 James Robertson Parkway, Nashville, Tenn., 37219

Texas Association for Mental Health, 103 Lantern Lane, Austin, Texas, 78731

Utah Association for Mental Health, 1370 S.W. Temple, Salt Lake City, Utah, 84115

Mental Health Association in **Virginia**, Suite 203, 1806 Chantilly St., Richmond, Va., 23230

West Virginia Association for Mental Health, 702½ Lee St., Charleston, W. Va., 25301

Wisconsin Association for Mental Health, P.O. Box 1486, Madison, Wis., 53701

Index

age:
   cancer, **94-95, 122, 124-125**
   heart attack, **6, 12**
   stroke, **136**
alcohol, **20, 55, 73-74, 137-139**
American Cancer Society, **78-79, 81-82, 84, 94, 96, 107-111, 119, 122-125, 127, 142**
   list of state units, **145-148**
American Health Foundation, **115**
American Heart Association, **8, 17, 20-24, 45-46, 61-63, 66, 68**
   list of state units, **142-145**
American Red Cross, **68**
Ames, Dr. Bruce N., **106**
Anderson, Grace, **131-134**
animal tests, **76, 103-107**
asbestos, **76, 108-110**
Ashman, Patricia, **21**
aspirin, **134-135**

Baker, Dr. A. B., **132-136**
benzo(a)pyrene, **112**
birth control pill, **36, 98**
Blackburn, Dr. Henry, **8-9, 12, 16-20, 52, 54**
bladder cancer, **75, 82, 104-105, 121**
blood pressure, **5-11, 13, 25-32, 129**
brain, **10, 13, 66-67, 129, 132-136**
breast cancer, **70-71, 74, 76, 93-95, 100, 115-117, 119-122, 125, 127** *(see also mammography)*
breast self-examination, **119, 122, 127, 138**
Byron, Rep. Goodloe, **45**

CPR (cardio-pulmonary resuscitation), **65-68, 142**
Campion, Dr. Brian, **61-62**
Canada, **137-140**
cancer, **1, 11, 71; Chapters 10-15; 137**
   chemical causes, **75-78, 103-114**
   early detection, **119-127**
   medical-related causes, **93-102**
   role of diet, **115-118**
   smoking, **79-91**
   symptoms, **125-127**
   See separate listings for various type of cancer, such colon, skin, breast cancer, etc.

Cancer Information Service, **142, 148-149**
carbon monoxide, **6, 11, 33-35**
cardio-pulmonary resuscitation, **65-68, 142**
carotid artery, **132-134**
cells, **71, 120-121**
Center for Disease Control, **81**
cervical cancer, **94, 99, 119, 123**
Changing Weighs, **37, 40**
charcoal broiling, **112**
cholesterol, **5-10, 13, 15-24, 28, 39, 47, 115-118, 129, 137**
cigar, **35, 138**
cigarettes *(see smoking)*
Clark, Kenneth, **59-61**
Clark, Nick, **33-35**
Clark, Dr. R. Lee, **81**
cleaning fluids, **112**
Cobb, Dr. Leonard, **67**
colon, cancer of (including adjoining rectum), **70-71, 74, 76-77, 108, 115-117, 119, 121-123, 125**
Consumer Product Safety Commission, **109**
Cornell University, **53**
coronary artery, **2-3, 5-6, 15, 17, 19, 28, 34, 53-54, 60, 116, 129**

DES (diethylstilbestrol), **93-94, 99-100**
death, leading causes of, **1, 141**
dental X-rays, **96-97, 101**
diabetes, **1, 11, 39, 137**
Dickinson College, **101**
diet and cancer, **74, 115-118**
diet and heart attacks, **15-24**
diethylstilbestrol (DES), **93-94, 99-100**
drugs, **19, 26, 93, 98, 138-139**
dyes, food, **112**
dyes, hair, **113**

early warning signs of cancer, **125-126**
eggs, **6, 10, 16, 21-22**
emphysema, **1, 8, 36, 137**
endometrial cancer, **97-98, 124**
Enstrom, Dr. James E., **76**
esophagus, cancer of, **74, 82, 108, 125**
estrogen, **93, 97-98**
exercise, **5-7, 11-12, 18, 39-40, 45-50, 137**

fibers, **115-117**
Finland, **16**

fluorocarbons, **113-114**
fluoroscope, **102**
Food and Drug Adminstration, **36, 93, 96-97, 104, 113**
Framingham, Mass., Heart Study, **7-8**
Frederick, Morris, **131-134**
Friedman, Dr. Meyer, **52-54, 56**
fungicides, **111-112**

garden and lawn chemicals, **111-112**
Garrison, Frank, **65-67**
genetic (heredity), **13, 18, 77**
Gilbertsen, Dr. Victor, **120-123, 125**

HDL (high-density lipoprotein), **15-21, 39, 47**
hair dryers, **109**
hair dyes, **113**
Hall, Dr. Robert, **10**
Halvorsen, Daniel, **39-40**
hamburgers, **112-113**
Hammond, Dr. E. Cuyler, **82, 108-109**
Harvard University, **46**
Health and Welfare Canada, **139-40**
Health Research Group, **102, 106**
heart, basic workings of, **3**
heart attacks, **1, 3; Chapters 1-9; 115-116, 129, 137**
   blood pressure as risk factor, **25-31**
   diet as risk factor, **15-24,**
   exercise as risk factor, **45-50**
   explanation of, **3**
   prevention overview, **5-13**
   smoking as risk factor, **33-36**
   stress as risk factor, **51-57**
   symptoms, **59-63**
   weight as risk factor, **37-44**
   what to do in case of, **59-68**
heredity, **13, 18, 77**
high blood pressure *(see blood pressure)*
high-density lipoprotein (HDL), **15-21, 39, 47**
Hinkle, Dr. Lawrence, **54**
Holleb, Dr. Arthur, **94**
hormones, **6, 12, 16, 53, 93, 117** *(see also DES, estrogen)*
Horn, Dr. Daniel, **80, 82-84, 87**
Hurley, Jim, **65-66**
Hurwitz, Dr. Paul, **25**
hypertension *(see high blood pressure)*

Israel, 36, 116

Jacoves, Richard, 51, 54
Japan, 8-9, 52-53, 77, 94, 115-116
Jesse, Dr. Mary Jane, 27-28
jogging *(see exercise)*

Kannel, Dr. William, 5-6, 8-9, 20
Kennedy, Dr. Donald, 104-105
kidney cancer, 75-76, 82
kidney disease, 25

Laboratory of Physiological Hygiene, 8, 12, 16, 39, 49
larynx, cancer of, 82, 121
Laws, Priscilla, 101-102
Leclair, Hank, 140
leukemia, 70, 96, 102
lifestyle quiz, 137-140
Lilja, Dr. Patrick, 67
liver cancer, 75
low blood pressure, 30
lung cancer, 8, 70-71, 74, 76-77, 79, 81, 105, 121, 124-125
lymphoma, 70-71

mammography (breast X-rays), 94-95, 120
Mayo Clinic, 96
melanoma, 111
menopause, 93, 97
Mental Health Association, 51, 56-57, 142
  list of state units, 149-151
mesothelioma, 108
Metropolitan Medical Center, 37, 40
Minnesota Poll, 81
Mitchell, Dr. Jere, 46-47
mole, 111, 125
Mondale, Walter, 25-26
Mormons, 76
Mount Sinai Hospital, Minneapolis, 132, 135
Mount Sinai Hospital, New York, 74, 103, 108-109
mouth, cancer in, 74, 82, 121, 125-126
Mullenbach, Vikki, 37

National Cancer Institute, 74, 76, 78, 80, 82, 87, 93-96, 98-100, 107, 110, 112-113, 115, 117, 121, 126, 142, 148
National Heart, Lung and Blood Institute, 5, 20, 25-27, 29
National Institute of Environmental Health Sciences, 104

Newell, Dr. Guy R., **117**
nicotine, **6, 11, 33-35**
nitrites, **112**
North Memorial Medical Center, **67**
Northwestern University, **53**

occult-blood test, **122-123**
oral cancer (mouth and throat), **70, 74, 82, 121, 125-126**
ovary, cancer of, **70, 124**
ozone, **114**

Pafenbarger, Dr. Ralph, **46**
paint thinners, **112**
pancreas, cancer of, **70, 82**
Pap test, **99, 119, 123-4, 126**
pesticides, **111-112**
pipe, **35, 138**
polyps, **122**
proctoscope (procto), **119, 122-123, 126**
prostate cancer, **70, 76, 121, 124-125**

Rall, Dr. David P., **104**
Rauscher, Dr. Frank, **73, 78, 96, 107-108, 119-120**
Richmond, Dr. Julius, **83**
Rosenman, Dr. Ray, **52-54, 56**
Rotman, Eileen, **33-35, 80-81, 83**

saccharin, **104-106**
St. Paul-Ramsey Medical Center, **61**
salt, **10-11, 26-28, 30**
Schneiderman, Dr. Marvin, **74-75, 98, 115**
Seattle, **67**
Selikoff, Dr. Irving, **73-74, 77, 103, 107-109**
Seventh Day Adventists, **116**
sexual habits, **74**
skin cancer, **70-71, 75, 110-111, 125**
smoking, **1, 137-138**
  cancer, **73-75, 77, 79-84, 105, 110, 124**
  heart disease, **5-8, 11, 18, 33-36, 48, 53**
  stroke, **129**
solvent cleaners, **112**
Stamler, Dr. Jeremiah, **53**
stilbestrol *(see DES)*
stomach cancer, **108, 125**
stress, **1, 5-6, 12, 48, 51-57, 86, 142**
stroke, **1, 9-10, 13, 25, 129, 131-137**

sun, **73, 75, 103, 110-111**
symptoms:
　cancer, **125-127**
　heart attack, **59-63**
　stroke, **131-136**

TIA (transient ischemic attack), **135**
tar, cigarette, **33-35, 74, 82-83**
teen-age smoking, **79-80, 84**
tension *(see stress)*
Texas Heart Institute, **10**
thyroid cancer, **93, 95-96, 100-101**
transient ischemic attack, **135**
triglycerides, **18**
Tris, **76, 106**
type A (or B) behavior, **52-56**

ultraviolet rays, **110-111**
University of California, **52, 106**
University of California at Los Angeles, **76**
University of Minnesota, **8, 12, 16, 21, 34, 39, 49, 52, 54, 80, 120**
University of Texas Cancer Center, **81**
University of Texas medical school, Dallas, **46**
Unsmoke, **34, 80**
Upton, Dr. Arthur, **82, 96-97, 100, 112-113**
uterus, cancer of the, **70, 76, 93-94, 97-99, 119, 121, 123-125** *(see also separate listings for cervical and endometrial cancer)*

Ward, Graham, **26, 29-31**
wart, **111, 125**
Washington University, **112**
weight, **1, 5-6, 11, 18, 26, 30, 37-44, 48, 137**
Witte, Dr. John, **81**
Wolfe, Dr. Sidney, **106**
Women:
　heart attacks, **6, 12**
　smoking, **36**
Wynder, Dr. Ernst L., **115**

X-rays, **73, 75, 93-97, 100-102**

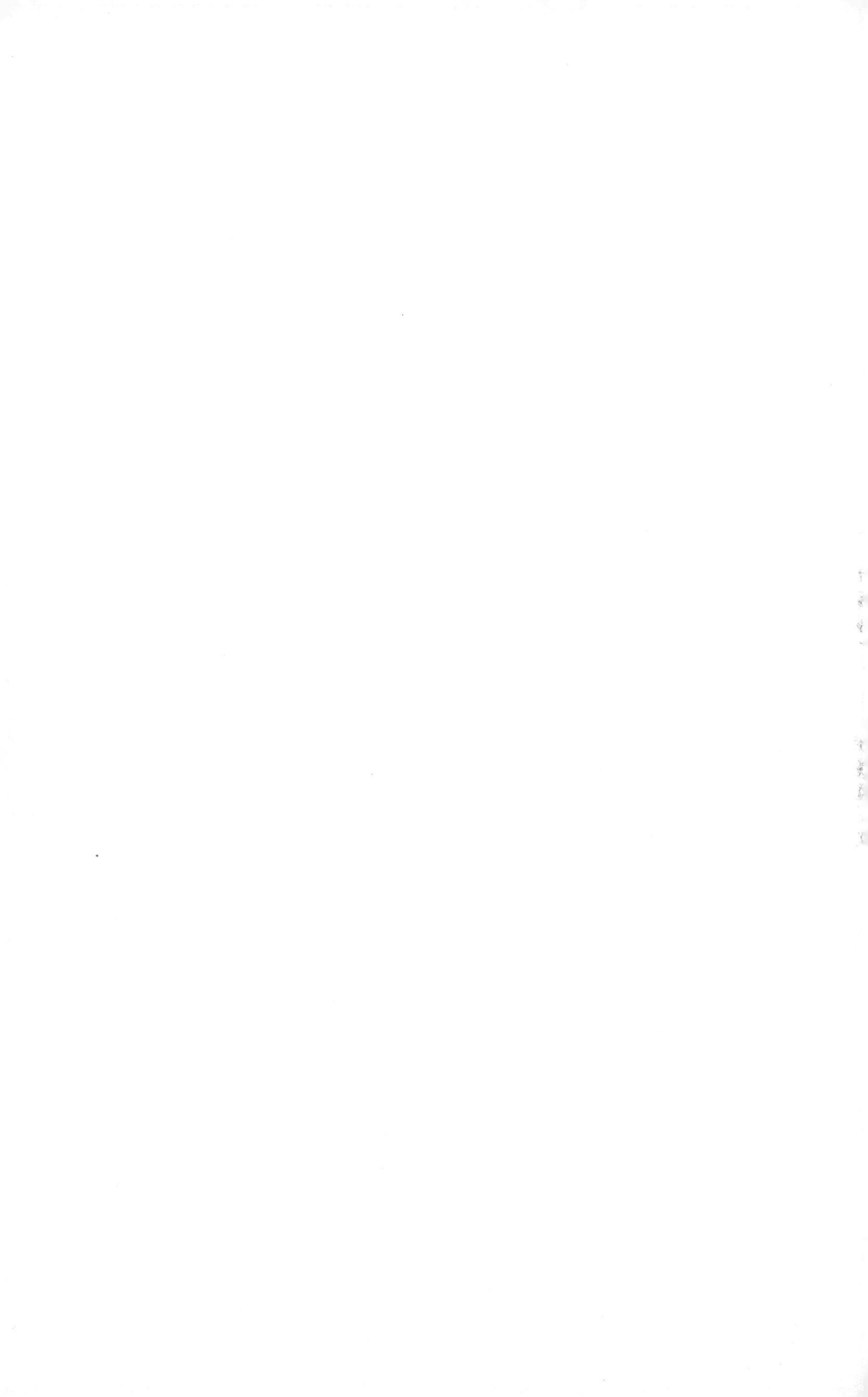

Heart attack signals

You should know these symptoms of a possible heart attack:

■ Typically there is uncomfortable pressure, fullness, squeezing or pain in the center of the chest (behind the breastbone) lasting two minutes or more.

■ Pain may — but doesn't always — spread to the shoulders, arm, neck or jaw.

■ Severe pain, dizziness, fainting, sweating, nausea or shortness of breath may also occur. But again, these symptoms aren't always present.

■ Sometimes the symptoms subside, then return. They aren't always severe.

■ Momentary sharp, stabbing twinges of pain usually are not signals of a heart attack.

What to do:

■ Sit down or, if you feel faint, lie down.

■ If the symptoms last two minutes or longer, assume that it may be a heart attack until a professional medical person says otherwise.

Emergency telephone numbers:

Emergency service
[Rescue squad, ambulance, etc.]

Name ⎯⎯⎯⎯⎯⎯⎯⎯⎯⎯⎯⎯⎯⎯⎯⎯⎯⎯⎯⎯⎯⎯⎯⎯⎯⎯⎯

Phone ⎯⎯⎯⎯⎯⎯⎯⎯⎯⎯⎯⎯⎯⎯⎯⎯⎯⎯⎯⎯⎯⎯⎯⎯⎯⎯

Physician

Name ⎯⎯⎯⎯⎯⎯⎯⎯⎯⎯⎯⎯⎯⎯⎯⎯⎯⎯⎯⎯⎯⎯⎯⎯⎯⎯⎯

Phone ⎯⎯⎯⎯⎯⎯⎯⎯⎯⎯⎯⎯⎯⎯⎯⎯⎯⎯⎯⎯⎯⎯⎯⎯⎯⎯

Give your precise address or location. Say that a heart attack is suspected. If you're calling for someone who is unconscious and not moving, say a cardiac arrest is suspected.

(Perforated for removal from book and posting in home, office, etc. If more copies are needed, use photocopying machine.)

Heart attack signals

You should know these symptoms of a possible heart attack:

■ Typically there is uncomfortable pressure, fullness, squeezing or pain in the center of the chest (behind the breastbone) lasting two minutes or more.

■ Pain may — but doesn't always — spread to the shoulders, arm, neck or jaw.

■ Severe pain, dizziness, fainting, sweating, nausea or shortness of breath may also occur. But again, these symptoms aren't always present.

■ Sometimes the symptoms subside, then return. They aren't always severe.

■ Momentary sharp, stabbing twinges of pain usually are not signals of a heart attack.

What to do:

■ Sit down or, if you feel faint, lie down.

■ If the symptoms last two minutes or longer, assume that it may be a heart attack until a professional medical person says otherwise.

Emergency telephone numbers:

Emergency service
[Rescue squad, ambulance, etc.]

Name _____

Phone _____

Physician

Name _____

Phone _____

Give your precise address or location. Say that a heart attack is suspected. If you're calling for someone who is unconscious and not moving, say a cardiac arrest is suspected.

(Perforated for removal from book and posting in home, office, etc. If more copies are needed, use photocopying machine.)